6 STEPS *to a* STRONGER, PAIN-FREE BODY AND MIND

A Physiotherapist's Guide to Healing Back, Neck, and Body Pain, Reducing Stress, and Rebuilding Strength Through Simple Daily Movement

TINA BERCIC

Disclaimer

This book is intended for educational and informational purposes. It is not a substitute for professional medical advice, diagnosis, or treatment. Always seek the advice of your physician or other qualified health provider before beginning any new exercise program or making changes to your current pain management routine. The author and publisher assume no responsibility for any injury or adverse effects that may result from the use of the information contained in this book. Individual results may vary. Chronic pain can have multiple causes, and what works for one person may not work for another. If you experience severe or worsening pain, stop the exercises and consult a healthcare professional.

Edited by Fatima H. (Petrichoreditors.com)
Cover design by Libro Valorem Publishing
Interior layout by Libro Valorem Publishing

Hardcover ISBN: 978-961-97401-0-1
Paperback ISBN: 978-961-97401-1-8
Ebook ISBN: 978-961-97401-2-5

Cataloguing-in-Publication (CIP) record prepared by the National and University Library in Ljubljana
Kataložni zapis o publikaciji (CIP) pripravili v Narodni in univerzitetni knjižnici v Ljubljani
COBISS.SI-ID 274237443

First Edition: 2026
Self-published by Tina Bercic
Print on Demand
Izola, Slovenia

Dedication

To everyone enduring long-term suffering and feeling overlooked. This book aims to offer understanding, reveal your resilience, and provide meaningful guidance for reclaiming your life and well-being. It is dedicated to the calm strength that comes from not giving up and the deep wisdom that comes from a body that has learned to show its needs through pain. May you discover peace, renewed strength, and a deeper awareness of your capabilities. With sincere respect, I wish you recovery.

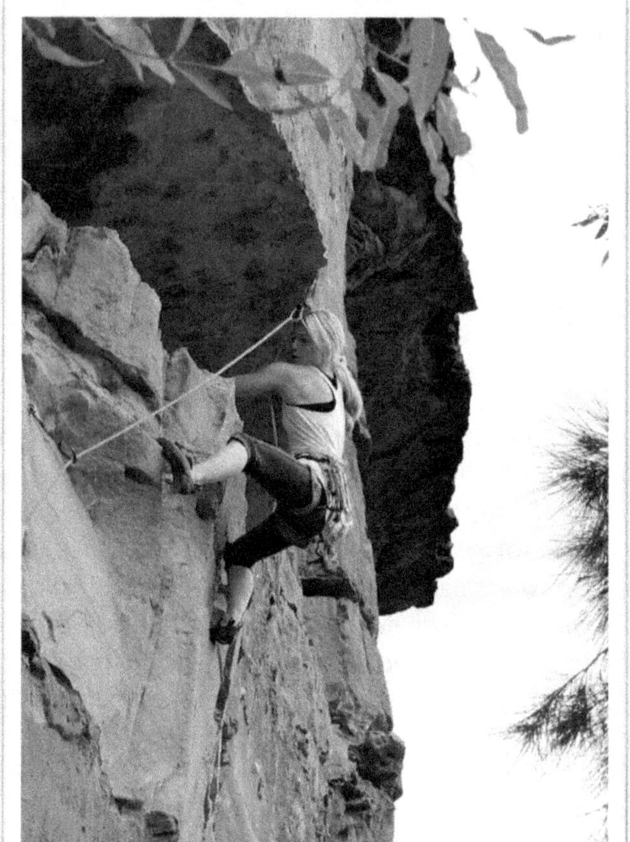

Blue Mountains, Australia

Dedication

To everyone enduring long-term suffering and feeling overlooked. This book aims to offer understanding, reveal your resilience, and provide meaningful guidance for reclaiming your life and well-being. It is dedicated to the calm strength that comes from not giving up and the deep wisdom that comes from a body that has learned to show its needs through pain. May you discover peace, renewed strength, and a deeper awareness of your capabilities. With sincere respect, I wish you recovery.

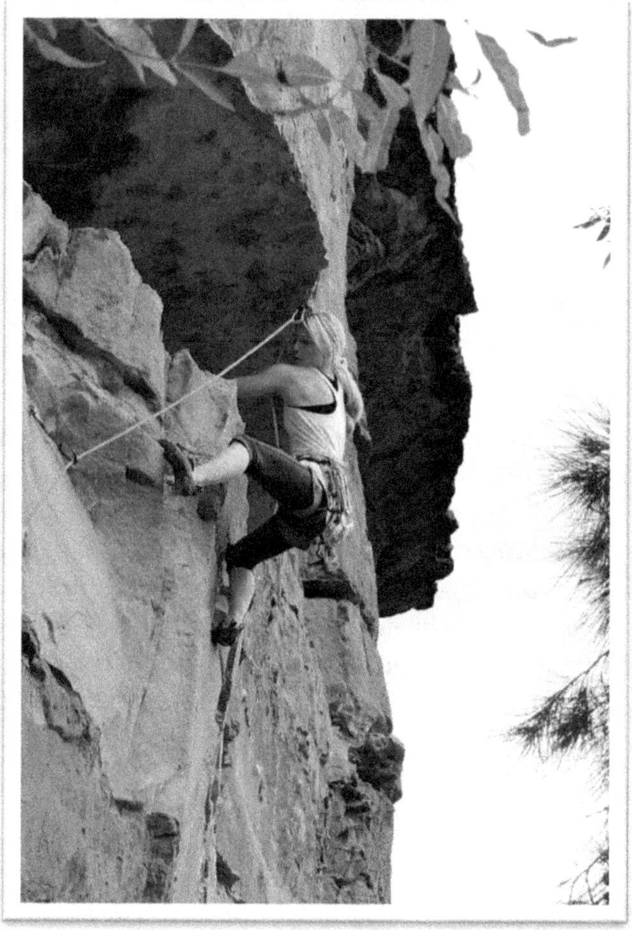

Blue Mountains, Australia

About the Author

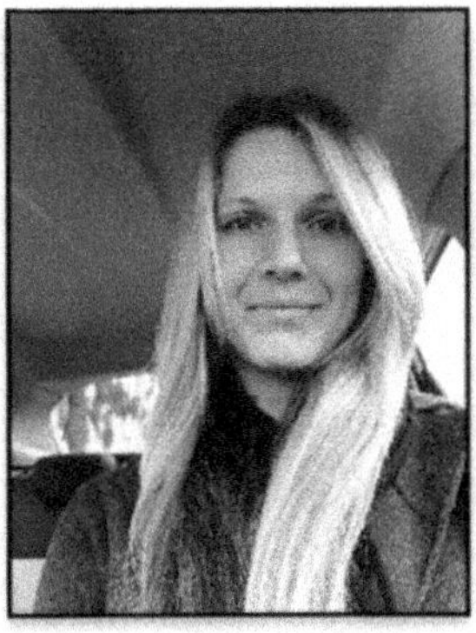

Tina Bercic is a licensed physiotherapist, certified yoga teacher, and climber who has spent years working with people experiencing chronic pain. She trained in physiotherapy with a focus on musculoskeletal rehabilitation and has since integrated principles from yoga, neuroscience, and pain science into her clinical practice. Through her work in Slovenia and internationally, she has helped clients move beyond structural explanations of pain and discover how nervous system regulation, movement variability, and self-awareness can lead to lasting relief. When she's not treating clients or teaching, Tina can be found on climbing routes, where she continues to learn how the mind and body adapt under pressure.

Praise for the Book

"It's not very often that you get practical, trustworthy advice from experts who not only excel in their fields, but also embody what's possible through consistent practice and discipline. This book brings together the perfect combination of an athlete and a physiotherapist, so you know the guidance isn't just theoretically sound, but tested, lived, and necessary in their own daily routines.

As someone who has dealt with chronic upper-back pain from long hours of sitting and working, I found this guide genuinely helpful. It introduced me to simple exercises that actually work. I highly recommend Tina's book to anyone experiencing chronic pain, tension, or restlessness, especially if you're unsure where to start. This guide walks you through everything with clarity and care."

— ***Fatima H., Developmental and Line Editor***

"This book changed my understanding of pain by showing me how emotions like stress, along with long-term habits such as lack of sleep and inadequate diet, amplify it. The author's approach is super compassionate and real; she doesn't sugarcoat it but helps readers understand what's going on. The best part is that she caters to everyone's needs by providing alternatives. It's a game-changer if you're looking for relief and a more mindful approach to your body."

— ***Ayesha M., Manager***

"Working in the IT sector, I spend long hours sitting, often under constant cognitive load and deadlines, which over time has led to persistent neck stiffness and low-level chronic discomfort. Since I personally know Tina and am aware of her extensive experience as a physiotherapist, I had a high level of trust in her approach from the start—and the book fully reflects her knowledge, professionalism, and real-world expertise.

What I appreciated most is that the book doesn't just focus on "fixing posture" or prescribing generic exercises; it clearly explains why the body feels the way it does, especially through the role of stress and the nervous system. That perspective was incredibly helpful for me.

It offers a practical way of dealing with chronic pain while being easy to incorporate into my daily routine. Exercises are simple yet effective; they helped me become more aware of how tension builds throughout the day. Over time, I've noticed great progress not only in my posture and well-being, but also in my mental clarity. I would highly recommend this book to anyone in a similar line of work looking for a realistic and sustainable way to manage pain and stress. "

— ***Anze N., Senior Software Engineer***

"What I really like about the author is that she does not chase perfection. She pushes back against the idea of perfect posture and instead explains why movement variety and body awareness matter far more. That change alone helped me stop overthinking how I sit and start paying attention to how I actually feel.

For anyone who has chronic pain, tension that never fully goes away, restlessness you can't explain, or simply a body that feels older than it should, this book is a genuine resource. It is compassionate without being preachy, practical without being rigid, and thorough without being overwhelming. The author brings together physiotherapy, yoga, climbing, and neuroscience in a way that feels clear and grounded.

I came to this book looking for relief, but what I found was understanding. And from that understanding, I finally started to heal. That's what a truly good book does—it doesn't just tell you what to do; it changes how you see yourself. This one did exactly that for me."

— ***Dr. Joshua O., Editor***

Table of Contents

Table of Contents

INTRODUCTION

Why Stress Makes Your Pain Worse and How You Can Stop It

Chronic pain is shaped by more than what happens in the body. Stress, sleep, emotions, movement, and daily life can all influence how pain is experienced.

Living with chronic pain feels disorienting. Activities that once felt effortless now provoke tension or apprehension. Sitting at a desk, turning your head, and bending to tie your shoes can all become sources of fear. Pain changes how you think, move, and plan your day. For many people, the most exhausting part is the persistent uncertainty. Why does the pain persist? Why is there no clear explanation? Why do treatments fail to provide lasting relief?

For years, I saw this confusion from both sides of the treatment table. As a physiotherapist, I helped people who had done everything they were told to do. They strengthened their "weak" muscles, stretched their "tight" ones, fixed their posture, rested when told to, and pushed through when told to, but the pain kept coming back. As a yoga teacher, I saw the same people relax, breathe, and move easily in one setting, then tighten up and hurt again in different environments. As a climber, I learned how much the mind and nervous system affect how well the body moves, adapts, and heals.

What I couldn't ignore any longer was this: pain isn't just a problem with tissue. In fact, stress plays a significant role in how chronic pain begins, worsens, and persists.[1] Recognizing this connection is crucial, as it allows us to see the multifaceted nature of pain.

Therefore, this book is designed to help you understand that connection in real life, guiding you through practical strategies to address both stress and pain. By applying the insights offered within these pages, you'll learn how to start breaking the cycle of pain today. Through a combination of understanding, consistency, and daily movement, you can take meaningful steps towards relief and improved well-being.

How I Learned to See Pain Differently

When I first trained as a physiotherapist, I was taught to look for mechanical problems. We assessed joints, muscles, posture, and movement patterns. Pain was assumed to be the result of something "wrong" in the body: something weak, tight, degenerated, or misaligned. So, we had to find the broken part and fix it. This model works well for acute injuries—a broken bone, a torn ligament, or a recent trauma requires structural care. But with experience, I began to notice how poorly this model explained chronic pain. I've seen people whose scans revealed bulging discs, arthritis, or so-called "flaws" in their posture, yet they moved freely without pain. Conversely, I've also encountered individuals whose imaging appeared completely normal, but they lived with persistent discomfort. These contrasting experiences highlight a crucial point: research consistently shows a disconnect between the tissue damage visible on clinical imaging and the actual symptoms patients report.

I also saw patterns that had little to do with anatomy. People's pain got worse when they were stressed, didn't get enough sleep, were under work pressure, or went through big life changes. Their symptoms changed daily, sometimes hourly, even though they weren't doing anything different. Exercises that were fine one week became painful the next, even though nothing had changed structurally. My own experiences confirmed these observations. Climbing requires presence and focus. When you're worried, or your mind is racing, your grip tightens, your breathing shortens, and your movements become less effective. When you're calm and focused, strength comes without effort. Yoga taught me something similar: you can't force flexibility and control. They happen when the nervous system feels safe enough to allow them.

This realization pointed to the missing link in most pain treatments: the nervous system. It regulates muscle tone, pain sensitivity, coordination, and recovery as a tangible, trainable physiological system. So, when I started using nervous system regulation, both with clients and handling my own climbing injuries, the results changed. Movement improved, but the bigger change was a growing sense of safety in the body. I experienced that shift myself. When the system felt calmer, pain no longer had to be loud, and progress happened in ways that strength alone had never produced.

The Outdated Story We've Been Told About Pain

Most people think that pain is a direct sign of injury. This belief is strengthened by scary imaging reports, dramatic language, and well-meaning advice that makes the body seem weak. Words like "degeneration," "wear and tear," "instability," and "bad posture" all imply that something is wrong with you and that it may not be fixable.

However, pain can continue even with safe tissue loads. When chronic pain has mechanical characteristics, it may signal early warning signs from a sensitized nervous system rather than a direct threat to tissues.[2] Pain clearly protects you when you have an acute injury. But when stress persists, the nervous system can remain on high alert even after tissues have healed.[3] In effect, the pain volume knob stays turned up. Movements that are safe for the structure start to feel dangerous, and activities that once used to be neutral now make you feel scared. This doesn't mean the pain is all in your head. It means your nervous system has become too protective. Just as it learned to amplify danger signals, it can also learn a new, healthier pattern—one that restores safety and reduces unnecessary pain.

Stress, Sedentary Living, and a Nervous System that Never Switches Off

The human nervous system faces many challenges in modern life. We are always being stimulated, getting too much information, feeling rushed, and sitting for long periods, often all at once. Stress activates the sympathetic nervous system, the fight-or-flight response. This state prepares the body for action by tightening muscles, altering breathing, and increasing pain sensitivity. This response is helpful in short bursts, but when it happens repeatedly, it causes problems.

Your muscles stay slightly contracted all day. Breathing becomes shallow and less efficient, limiting oxygen exchange and keeping the system in a heightened state. Recovery processes slow down, and movement loses its natural fluidity. Instead of adapting smoothly, the body begins to move cautiously. Over time, this constant low-level tension starts

to feel normal; however, it continues to place ongoing strain on both tissues and the nervous system.[4] Compounding this issue, inactivity worsens it. When the body remains stationary, tension builds as it fails to move through a wide range of motion. Consequently, the nervous system receives fewer signals, indicating that movement is safe and manageable. As a result, the body increasingly feels stiff and reactive, making it harder to trust in its ability to move freely.

Why "Pushing Through" Rarely Works

When people are in pain, they sometimes try harder. They push through pain, force stretches, or work hard to strengthen muscles to regain control. Some people, however, do the opposite, not moving at all because they're afraid of making things worse. Both answers make sense, but they often don't work. When movement is performed in a state of threat, the nervous system interprets it as evidence of danger.[5] As muscles become tighter, pain sensitivity increases. Consequently, the body begins to associate movement with danger.

This is why so many people say, "Exercise helps for a while, but then my pain comes back." The stress response that caused the problem was never addressed. The nervous system never learned that it was safe to let go. To really change, you need a different approach. You need to prioritize movement variety over load, awareness over intensity, and consistency over effort.

A Different Framework for Healing

The main idea of this book is simple: the nervous system must feel safe enough for pain relief to last, and movement is a way to communicate with it. When movement is slow, controlled, and planned, it signals that everything is safe. If you do it repeatedly, it retrains the system to downregulate. This doesn't mean you should avoid strength or challenge. It means putting them in the right order. Thus, calm comes before capacity, and regulation comes before resilience. Over time, I developed this knowledge into a simple, repeatable system called **the 6-Step Method**.

The Six-step Method: An Overview

Each step builds on the last, working on pain from the inside out.

- **Step 1: Calm the nervous system**. This reduces baseline stress and pain sensitivity. It's the foundation for the entire method.
- **Step 2: Regain body awareness**. You learn to feel safe rather than scared as you experience sensations again. This focuses on sensory awareness and emotional reconnection with the body.
- **Step 3: Release chronic muscle tension**. This addresses tension gently without forcing muscles to stretch.
- **Step 4: Improve alignment and stability**. This promotes dynamic alignment without rigid posture corrections, allowing for more natural movement patterns.
- **Step 5: Build strength gradually**. This develops confidence in movement and helps you trust your body again.
- **Step 6: Integrate changes into daily life**. This ensures the practices become a regular part of your routine, promoting lasting change.

These steps work together to create a process that adapts to your body and your life.

Who This Book is Written For

This book is for people who have chronic pain and want to understand what is happening in their bodies. It is for people who feel tense, on edge, or disconnected and think that stress is a bigger part of their symptoms than they have been told. It's for people who want to move without fear of hurting themselves.

You don't have to be fit, flexible, or know how to do yoga. You don't have to get rid of the pain before you start. You just need to be curious about your body rather than judgmental.

What You Can Expect

This book doesn't offer quick fixes or miracle cures. Healing doesn't always happen in a straight line, and pain isn't something you fight to get rid of. This book provides practical tools and a framework for change that unfolds over time. Change takes time, discipline, and consistency.

By the end of this book, you will have a different understanding of your pain. You will learn how stress and your thoughts affect your body and nervous system. You'll learn simple, effective ways to calm that system down and move more easily. You will start to get stronger and more resilient without being afraid. Most importantly, you won't feel lost in your own body anymore.

You will understand your pain, learn how stress, beliefs, and mental state affect your health. Pain is real. It's part of life. But suffering doesn't have to be permanent. You will soothe your nervous system using simple, effective stress management techniques. You will move with freedom and discover confidence in movement.

The Starting Point

This is the beginning of your journey. You'll look at pain in a new way and work toward a more balanced life. We will explore ways to reduce stress, reconnect with your body's natural wisdom, and build a strong foundation for living with less pain and more energy. Healing is about changing how you relate to your body and your pain.[6]

This book isn't about avoiding pain. It's about learning to process pain and navigate it with less resistance. We will work together to help you become calmer, stronger, and more capable so you can live a fuller life.

By the end of this book, you will have gained a deeper understanding of your pain, learned to regulate your nervous system, and achieved greater freedom of movement. This change comes from building real understanding.

This is the starting point of your journey.

CHAPTER 1

Calm the System

Pain is not simply a signal of tissue damage, but a protective output of the nervous system shaped by context, perception, and past experience.

Research shows that more than 85% of low back pain cases cannot be reliably attributed to a specific disease or spinal abnormality.[1] This number hits people in two ways. On one hand, it's a relief, finally proof that what shows up on scans or tests doesn't fully explain their pain. But it's also scary because if nothing is obviously "wrong," where does the pain come from, and why does it feel so real? Understanding pain involves recognizing it as a mechanism through which the nervous system protects itself, rather than merely an indicator of tissue damage.[2] Pain functions as a form of information that can vary based on the context. It is influenced by various factors, including physical input, stress levels, emotional burdens, past experiences, and the brain's sense of safety.[3]

Pain can persist even when the body is structurally healthy, but the nervous system is overwhelmed by stress, fear, past experiences, and the constant effort to stay on guard.[4]

Therefore, this chapter is about the first and most important step in healing: calming your nervous system. Before you can rebuild strength or move without feeling stiff, the system that controls how we feel pain must be taken out of survival mode. Slowing your breathing, taking short breaks, or moving gently in ways that feel safe tells your body it can relax and does not need to stay tense. If you skip this part, any progress you make doesn't last long. It's like building a house on sand.

So, let's begin on this journey together.

The Hidden Relationship Between Stress and Muscle Tension

People don't often feel stress as a single event. It builds up slowly, becoming part of everyday life through responsibility, pressure, and constant stimulation. Stress is often talked about as a mental or emotional state, but its most obvious and consistent form is physical. When the nervous system perceives a threat, it increases muscle tone. This is called the fight-or-flight response. In this state, the brain prepares the body to act when it senses danger. Muscles contract to keep joints stable, protect important organs, and allow quick movement. Similarly, heart rate goes up, and breathing gets faster and shallower. Focus narrows as the brain prioritizes survival over clear thinking.[5]

This response is protective in the short term. The problem is when stress shifts from acute to chronic. In today's world, threats are often not physical or easy to deal with. Emails, deadlines, money problems, family issues, interpersonal stress, and the need to always do well don't seem to end. Hence, the nervous system never gets a message that it is safe to stop. As a result, muscles remain partially contracted long after the stressor has gone away. This contraction is often not noticeable, but it has big effects over time. When muscle tone stays the same, blood flow and oxygen delivery slow down, and the nerves around the area become more sensitive. Thus, what started out as protection slowly becomes discomfort, stiffness, and then pain.[6]

Over time, this constant state of contraction doesn't just affect circulation and nerve sensitivity; it begins to shape the body itself. The protective response that once served a purpose becomes ingrained in specific muscle groups, creating recognizable patterns of tension that reflect the body's bracing against ongoing stress.

Chronic stress has a big effect on some parts of the body. To protect the head and sensory organs, the neck and shoulders often tighten. The jaw tightens in preparation or restraint, which often causes headaches or pain in the temporomandibular joint.[7] The rib cage gets stiff, making it hard to breathe and keeping you alert. Hips bracing to keep the body stable can cause lower back or pelvic pain. These patterns are not random. They show how the body reacts to danger on its own. These protective patterns become automatic when stress is always there. Understanding these physiological responses helps to clarify the underlying trigger for such reactions, which brings us to the emotional component involved.

Emotional stress is at the heart of all this. Your nervous system doesn't distinguish between physical threats and emotional ones. Maybe it's an unresolved conflict, lingering grief, constant worry, or a feeling of being trapped in a tough situation. Your body reacts almost the same way it would if you were facing real danger.[8] Even when there is nothing to physically escape from, the body gets ready to deal with it.

In real life, pain often shifts depending on what's going on in your life, not just what you're doing physically. Think of a young professional working in a fast-paced office. During a quiet Sunday at home, she feels relaxed and notices no pain.

But once Monday arrives, the flood of emails, meetings, and deadlines triggers her nervous system. Her shoulders begin to creep upward toward her ears, her jaw clenches unconsciously, and her breathing becomes shallow. By Wednesday, she has a dull headache and stiffness in her neck. Nothing about her muscles or joints has physically changed since the weekend; the difference is that her body is bracing against the ongoing stress signals.

The pain isn't random; it's her nervous system staying "switched on" as if danger were still present. The tissues themselves haven't changed, but the nervous system is now more active. Once you see this, it's easier to stop blaming your body for what you're feeling and start noticing how it actually adapts. Your body isn't broken. It's just responding to ongoing stress the best way it can.

The Brain's Pain Alarm System and Fear-Pain Cycle

Modern science explains pain as the body's way of protecting itself. It's like an alarm system that sometimes goes overboard. Muscles, joints, and connective tissue transmit sensory information to the nervous system; however, the brain determines whether this information signifies danger. The brain figures out how much protection the body needs based on new sensory information, past experiences, emotional context, and perceived threat. [9] When the predicted threat is high, pain output increases to encourage caution, guarding, or avoidance.[10]

In this way, pain is not just a signal from the body; it's a prediction shaped by the brain. And when stress enters the picture, it amplifies those predictions, making the alarm system more sensitive and more likely to misfire.

When someone is stressed out, tired, or emotionally drained, their brain becomes more alert. It looks more closely for possible threats and makes it easier for pain to start. Movements that used to be okay may now seem dangerous. Feelings that used to be neutral can turn uncomfortable or scary. Once you have chronic pain, fear often makes it worse. You start to worry about when the pain will hit. You avoid activities that might trigger it. You tense up at the slightest hint of discomfort. This is all perfectly normal. Your brain is trying to keep you safe.

But here's what happens: when you're afraid of pain, your nervous system stays on high alert. It becomes more sensitive. It starts treating more things as dangerous. This creates what we call the fear-pain cycle.[11] You feel pain. Fear kicks in. The nervous system ramps up, and pain increases again. The cycle keeps going. This happens a lot with migraines and other conditions. People are afraid of getting another migraine. They avoid triggers. They constantly monitor their bodies for warning signs. That constant vigilance can actually make migraines happen more often.[12] The same thing happens with back pain, neck pain, fibromyalgia, and other chronic pain conditions. Breaking this cycle doesn't mean ignoring pain or pretending it doesn't hurt. It means teaching your brain that the pain signals aren't as dangerous as they feel.

This is why pain can be hard to predict and understand. One day, moving around feels easy and natural. The same movement makes you feel bad or scared the next day. Nothing "broke" while you slept. The context of the nervous system changed. Stress also makes it harder for the brain to determine whether something is safe. When the system is overloaded, it favors protection.[13] This bias keeps you alive.

However, when protection goes too far, pain lasts longer than it should.

Many people think this persistence means something is very wrong with their bodies. In fact, it is often proof that the nervous system has learned to stay on high alert. The good news is that this kind of learning can be undone. When the brain is repeatedly exposed to safe experiences, it can change how it makes predictions.[14]

Sedentary Life as a Stress Multiplier

People often perceive modern stress as primarily a mental challenge, but one of the most effective ways to exacerbate it is through inactivity. Long hours spent sitting, excessive screen time, and high cognitive demands create a situation in which our bodies remain mostly still, while our nervous systems are highly engaged. Our bodies have evolved to cope with stress through movement.[15] When we walk, adjust our posture, and utilize our breath in a full range of motion, we provide our nervous systems with valuable feedback that reinforces our strength, flexibility, and sense of safety. Without movement, stress has nowhere to dissipate.

From a mechanical perspective, prolonged inactivity can reduce tissue tolerance.[16] Regular movement is essential for maintaining healthy and well-lubricated joints.[17] To remain flexible and strong, muscles require a variety of movements, while connective tissue adapts positively to different types of loading. After sitting for a long time, the first movement, standing up, bending, or turning, can feel stiff or sharp, and the nervous system may read that sensation as danger. This is one reason why many people feel worse at the end of a day spent sitting still than after doing some light exercise. The stress isn't coming from work. It's coming from being still and from the nervous system always being active.

A sedentary lifestyle does more than just weaken the body. It amplifies stress signals, disrupts breathing patterns, and intensifies pain.[18] The nervous system stays ready, but it doesn't improve if it doesn't get to move, grow, and let go regularly. A study found that walking for more than 100 minutes per day was associated with a 23% lower risk of chronic low back pain compared with walking less than 78 minutes per day.[19]

Their backs weren't magically 'fixed.' Regular movement can provide repeated experiences that help build confidence in movement, while also supporting physical capacity. Larger epidemiological research also suggests that regular physical activity may help protect against low back pain.[20]

People often miss the little things that make our nervous system more sensitive because they aren't obvious right away. We might think a headache is caused by bad posture or a stiff neck from sleeping in an uncomfortable position, but we don't realize that a big reason is the constant low-level stress we've been under. Our bodies are built to keep us safe, and when they sense a long-term threat, they use methods that can, ironically, cause chronic pain. This protective response includes increased muscle tone, more sensitive nerve endings, and changes in how the brain processes pain signals. This means that for a lot of people with chronic pain, the problem isn't just damaged tissues. It's also a nervous system that is too sensitive and stuck in a pattern of feeling threatened.

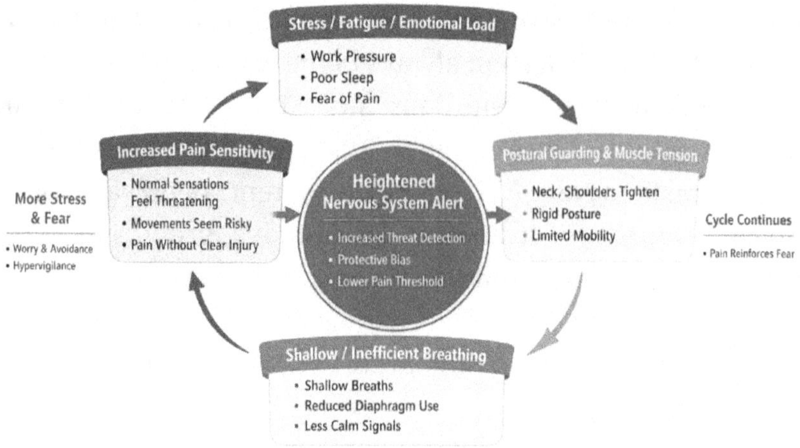

Figure 1.1: Diagram showing the relationship between stress, posture, breathing, and pain sensitivity.

Real People, Real Change

Recovery from chronic pain often feels impossible until you see it happen in real life. The following stories show how ordinary people, each with different struggles, rebuilt their lives by following a steady process rather than chasing quick fixes.

Laura, 55, dealt with chronic low-back pain and sciatica for almost ten years. She tried many treatments, like injections, massage, and seeing different specialists, but nothing helped for long. Finally, she joined a pain recovery program that focused on steady movement, learning about pain, and managing stress. She started with short walks and simple breathing exercises. After five months, she didn't need daily medication anymore. A year later, she was back to gardening, an activity she had stopped because of her pain.

Similarly, **Ethan, 41**, developed fibromyalgia after a car accident and was told he might never work full-time again. He began with ten minutes of gentle stretching each morning and started journaling about his emotions. He noticed his pain got worse when he felt powerless. Over the year, he rebuilt his routine. Now he runs a small business and sleeps well at night.

Maya, 34, had ongoing neck and shoulder pain that got worse when work was stressful. Scans didn't show any problems, but her pain was real. She joined a pain-coaching program that focused on slowly increasing movement, becoming more aware of her emotions, and calming her nervous system. As she became less afraid, her pain also lessened. After nine months, she stopped canceling plans with friends and finished her first yoga class in years.

They didn't discover a miracle cure; instead, they embraced a transformative journey grounded in a well-structured approach. By gaining a deeper understanding of pain, reducing fear, rebuilding safe movement, regulating their nervous systems, and fostering trust in their bodies, they each found a path to healing. Their stories remind us that lasting recovery is often a gradual process, shaped by perseverance and resilience. It's not about quick fixes, but rather about making consistent, meaningful changes that lead to a fulfilling life free from the limitations of chronic pain.

Why Traditional Pain Treatments Often Don't Work

Most traditional ways of dealing with pain focus on where the pain is felt, not on the system that causes it. Painkillers reduce acute pain, but they don't change how the brain sees danger. Massage may relax your muscles, but it doesn't teach your nervous system to stay relaxed. Heat can help with pain, but again, it doesn't address the underlying cause of your muscle tension. This is why relief often doesn't last. Many treatments only manage symptoms rather than solve the real problem. A lot of people go through the same thing: a treatment works for a little while, maybe a few hours or days, and then the pain comes back. Every time it happens again, it often feels worse than the last time. People start to think that they will always have to deal with pain.

Moreover, people rarely talk about how to regulate the nervous system. Most of us don't learn how to notice when our bodies are stressed, how to calm down after feeling threatened, or how to use movement and breathing to feel safe. Pain is often seen as something outside ourselves that needs fixing, rather than as a signal we can learn from and change. Even exercise-based treatments often miss this idea. When you feel threatened, your body's guarding response gets stronger.[21] Stretching too much can actually worsen this protective tension. It's important to know the difference between muscles that are tight from movement and those that are tight from protection. Without this understanding, people often push harder when their bodies actually need reassurance. This is where real change can begin.

Research over the past 20 years shows that ongoing pain and stiffness are rarely caused solely by tissue problems.[22] Studies on chronic back, neck, and general pain reveal that the brain changes how it senses and responds to threat and movement.[23] Even healthy tissues can feel tight or painful if the nervous system stays sensitive.[24]

When treatments merely relax muscles or provide temporary relief from symptoms, individuals may begin to feel reliant on constant interventions to manage their pain. Relief starts to feel like an external experience rather than something that can be sustained. Without retraining the nervous system to process movement and sensation calmly, stiffness is likely to return, as the protective patterns remain unchanged. For lasting relief, it's essential to show your body that it doesn't need to remain on high alert and that a sense of safety can be cultivated from within, rather than relying solely on external treatments.

Protective Versus Mechanical Stiffness

As a physiotherapist and yoga teacher, I have treated patients with both protective and mechanical stiffness. Addressing protective tension early is essential to prevent it from becoming counterproductive. If left unaddressed, protective tension can develop into chronic tightness that restricts movement, causes pain, and does not respond to traditional stretching or soft-tissue techniques such as massages, myofascial release therapy, and foam rolling.

To understand why traditional stretching or release techniques often fall short, it helps to look more deeply into the source of this stiffness. **Protective** stiffness originates from the nervous system rather than from damaged tissue. It's the body's way of communicating, "I'm uncertain about what's happening, so I'll limit movement as a precaution." This often occurs during periods of high stress, low-quality sleep, prolonged pain, or fear surrounding certain movements. Fortunately, protective stiffness often dissipates quickly when the nervous system feels more secure, sometimes simply through gentle movement, slower breathing, or redirecting focus away from the affected area. In contrast, **mechanical** stiffness typically requires a longer duration and repeated movement to alleviate.

But how can you tell whether your stiffness is protective rather than mechanical?

I would say always ask yourself, "Does this stiffness respond more to how I feel or to how much I move?"

If you have a hard time answering this, then I can give you a few indicators that can point out protective stiffness: A big red flag is when stretching makes areas feel worse. If you repeatedly stretch a tight region in your back or neck and only feel better for a short time before the discomfort comes back, your nervous system may be reacting to what it perceives as a threat, making you even more guarded.

If one side of your body is tense and doesn't respond to stretching on both sides, it could be a protective response. If only your right hip flexor feels tight even after stretching both sides equally, it could be because your nervous system is protecting that area for a reason, including an old injury that hasn't healed properly, joint instability, or weakness on that side.

Another clear sign is that the same regions keep tightening even when you stretch them often. If you've been stretching your hamstrings for months and not seeing any lasting results, the problem might not be that your muscles are too short but that your nervous system needs protection.

Painful stiffness that varies widely in intensity with stress levels, sleep quality, or mood also points to protective guarding.[25] Basic mechanical tightness develops when you move around a lot and goes away in a few days. Protective tension, on the other hand, lasts longer and changes with the general health of your nervous system.

Keep in mind that protective tension is a reflex of the nervous system, not just a problem with your muscles. The muscle often feels tight because it is overworked and exhausted, not because it is short. Traditional stretching can sometimes worsen things by inducing deep muscle lengthening, which may make your nervous system feel threatened.[26] To make your body feel comfortable enough to let go, you need a gentler, more holistic mind-body approach that considers your entire nervous system.[27] This will help you start to re-establish healthy movement patterns.

Breathing exercises, meditation, and walks in nature are all regular activities that can help your nervous system stay in balance. These activities can also help you relax and let go of protective tendencies.

Research suggests that pain can change how the trunk muscles are coordinated.[28] Rather than assuming your core is "weak," think of core stability exercises as an opportunity to gradually rebuild strength, coordination, and confidence in movement. For many people, improving trunk control becomes one useful part of returning to comfortable, everyday movement.

The quality of your sleep directly affects your nervous system's sensitivity to threats.[29] If you don't get enough sleep, your nervous system may become more sensitive, which might cause extra protective stress even when you're doing regular things.

Therefore, you need to shift your priorities if you want to make improvements that last. Your nervous system won't let your body heal or adapt until it feels safe. This is done through consistency and clarity, not force.

Your First Action Step: Reset the Stress-Pain Loop

Understanding how stress turns into pain is important, but understanding alone is not enough. The nervous system changes through experience, not just insight.[30] To start breaking the stress-pain cycle, the body needs to get clear, repeated signals that it is safe. You can't do this by forcing change or working really hard. Instead, you need to do simple, regular things that slowly take the system out of survival mode.

The goal of this first step is not to get rid of pain right away or make you more flexible. The real goal is to break the cycle of constant alertness that makes pain feel worse. When you practice these techniques regularly, even for just a few minutes, they can lower muscle tension, improve breathing and make your nervous system less likely to overreact to sensations.[31]

The following practices are designed to be easy to follow. They're for anyone who might already be in pain, feel nervous about moving, or worry that their body isn't strong enough. You shouldn't feel any strain, pain, or rush. If you do, just slow down or make the movement or breath gentler.

Healing begins when you feel safe.

The Three-Minute Grounding Breath

Breathing is an effective way to influence the nervous system. Slow, deep, and effortless breathing signals to the nervous system that the body is in a safe state.

To begin, select a position that provides comfort and stability, such as sitting in a chair with feet on the floor or lying on the back with knees bent and supported. The primary consideration is achieving a sense of stability and relaxation. Place one hand on the chest and the other on the lower ribs or abdomen. This contact is intended to enhance sensory feedback and awareness, not to control the breath. Inhale slowly through the nose, allowing the air to fill the rib cage and move gently into the abdomen. The chest should remain relaxed, without lifting or bracing. Exhale slowly through the mouth or nose to facilitate relaxation in the chest, ribs, and abdomen.

Try to let your exhale last a bit longer than your inhale. Breathing out for longer helps your body move from fight-or-flight mode to a state that supports healing and rest. As you breathe, notice where your body touches the ground. This feeling is important because your nervous system responds to these signs of support and grounding.

Continue this breathing pattern for approximately three minutes. If your mind starts to wander, gently redirect focus to the sensation of breath moving through the ribs and abdomen. There is no requirement to perform the breath perfectly. The intention is to facilitate ease. Many people report that this practice reduces pain or muscle tension. Even when it does not, it often leaves the body feeling less tense and more present. These subtle shifts are significant for pain regulation.

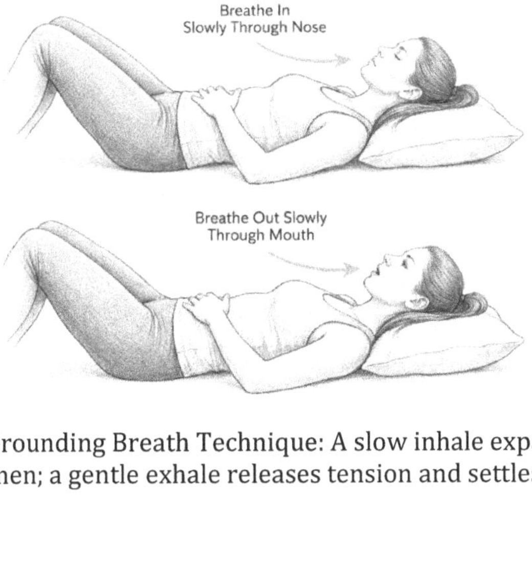

Figure 1.2: Grounding Breath Technique: A slow inhale expands the ribs and abdomen; a gentle exhale releases tension and settles the body.

The Mental Safety Cue

The nervous system is shaped by both physical stimuli and perceived meaning. [32] When the brain detects danger, it strengthens protective responses. When it perceives safety, these responses diminish. A mental safety cue can facilitate this process. While you continue to breathe calmly, try saying a short phrase that helps you feel safe. For example, you might say "I am safe right now" or "There is no rush right now." The idea isn't to force positive thinking or self-affirmation, but to find comfort in what feels true right now.

However, if a phrase feels awkward, pick something simpler or more neutral. If you quietly repeat the phrase, especially as you breathe out, your body can start to connect the words with a sense of relaxation. Practicing this regularly can help your nervous system react differently to what you feel inside. It's normal to feel uncomfortable, impatient, or doubtful at first. This often means you're used to being on alert. With practice, these feelings usually fade. You can use this mental safety cue anytime, but it's especially helpful when you're stressed or in pain. It serves as a reminder that not every sensation requires an immediate response or action.

Gentle Neck Mobility: Letting Go of Tension

Stress often leads to neck tension, as noted by Lundberg.[33] The neck is home to important sensory structures that play a crucial role in maintaining balance and alertness. [34] When stress strikes, you may experience stiffness in your neck, making movement difficult or even painful. This exercise isn't focused on stretching; rather, it gently reminds your nervous system that moving your neck is safe and can help relieve discomfort.

Try this exercise: Sit or stand so your spine feels supported. Let your shoulders relax and avoid forcing them down or back. Breathe slowly and steadily. Gently turn your head to the right, stopping before you feel any strain or pain. Keep the movement small at first. Pause and notice if you want to hold your breath or tense up. Then, slowly return to the center. Repeat on the left side, again stopping early and moving gently.

Switch sides for one to two minutes, focusing on how the movement feels rather than how far you can turn. The aim is to gradually release tension. As you begin to feel safer, you will notice that your neck moves more easily over time.

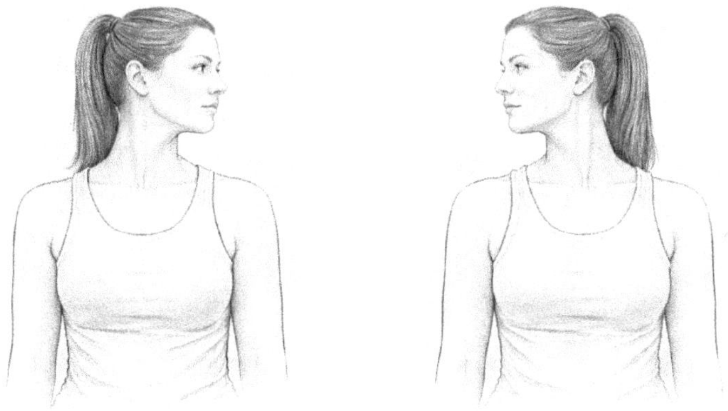

Figure 1.3: Gentle neck rotation within pain-free range

Rib Cage Mobility: Restoring Breath and Movement Variability

The rib cage plays a key role in both breathing and posture. If it gets stiff from stress or sitting too long, your breathing can become shallow, and your movement may feel tight.

Therefore, improving ribs and upper back mobility can help relax your muscles and make breathing easier.

Here's an exercise you can try: Sit or stand in a comfortable position. Rest your hands gently on the sides of your rib cage, just below your chest, or cross them over your chest. Keep your shoulders relaxed. As you breathe in, notice your ribs expanding. As you breathe out, let them soften inward. After a few breaths, start to add gentle movement.

Inhale and slowly turn your torso to the right. Stop if you feel any pain. Then, return to the center. Repeat on the left side in the same way. Keep your movements small, gentle, and relaxed, breathing naturally throughout.

Continue turning from side to side for 1 to 2 minutes, breathing normally. This isn't about fixing anything. It's about noticing how your spine moves. This exercise helps loosen up a part of the body that often gets stiff. It also helps connect your breathing and movement, which is important for your nervous system.

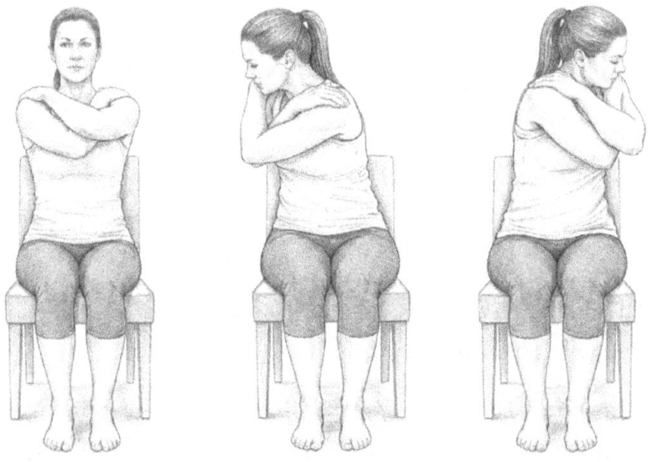

Figure 1.4: Rib cage rotation with hands crossed on the shoulder

Why These Simple Practices Matter

Many people don't realize how beneficial these practices can be. They aren't like regular workouts, and you might not notice results right away. Their gentle approach makes them effective. When you repeat these movements instead of pushing yourself, your nervous system can adapt. Calm breathing, moving without fear, and relaxing tension help your brain develop new habits.

Over time, your brain becomes more at ease. As your nervous system relaxes, your muscles loosen. Breathing gets easier, pain lessens, and movement feels safer. This helps your strength, flexibility, and resilience develop naturally.

You might find these methods helpful if you practice them regularly, even for a short time. Try one of these exercises today, even for just three to five minutes. Do them in the morning to start your day, in the evening to unwind, or during breaks to reduce stress.

Remember, these methods do not replace professional rehabilitation or medical care. They are meant to support your overall health.

A Shift in Perspective

Incorporating these effective practices into your routine can set the stage for a profound transformation in how you view your body and its capabilities. Rather than seeing your body as a source of pain or limitation, this new perspective encourages a relationship based on understanding and compassion.

This step can significantly alter people's perceptions of their bodies. Pain is a signal that we can learn from, not just something to be eliminated. Stress is a physical state that we can affect with small actions. The goal of calming the nervous system is not to permanently prevent issues. It's about helping your body regain its flexibility. Your body becomes stronger when it feels safe.

This is the foundation for everything else in this book.

In the next chapter, we'll discuss how to re-establish a connection with your body and increase your awareness. Learning to trust movement once more requires taking this crucial step. To truly change, you must be conscious. With it, you can turn your fear of movement into a source of confidence.

CHAPTER 2

Reconnect

Reconnecting with your body begins by noticing what you feel, without immediately judging, fearing, or trying to change it.

Disconnection has become a common issue in modern life, often more so than problems like weakness, stiffness, or poor posture. Many individuals find themselves disconnected from their bodies, moving through the day guided by screens, schedules, and constant mental activity. This disconnection often goes unnoticed until physical discomfort—such as a stiff neck, aching back, or sudden pain—forces us to pay attention to our bodies. For many, this moment is all too familiar. You might realize that your shoulders have crept up toward your ears for hours, your jaw feels tight, and your breathing has become shallow without your awareness of the change. The body has been signaling its discomfort for some time; pain is merely the volume turned up on these signals.

Moreover, living predominantly in the mind can lead to increased anxiety and stress. A continual fixation on the past or the future can lead to worry and fear. This mental overactivity often heightens stress levels, which in turn can manifest as physical pain.[1]

In practice, I've seen that restoring awareness often changes symptoms before strength or flexibility ever does. This chapter discusses how loss of body awareness can intensify pain and why restoring this connection is essential for healing.

But before improving movement, building strength, or relieving long-term tension, it is important to pay attention to your physical sensations. Awareness is not optional; it is necessary for meaningful change. Reconnecting isn't about searching for pain. It's about helping your brain interpret signals from your body more accurately. As this connection strengthens, movement becomes smoother, tension decreases, and pain often subsides.

Nervous System in the Chair Age

The human body evolved for diverse movement throughout the day, including walking, squatting, reaching, twisting, and frequent posture changes. As mentioned earlier, many people only engage in brief exercise periods between long stretches of sitting. Studies show that many adults now sit for 9 to 11 hours daily. [2] This prolonged inactivity has a significant impact on both the nervous and musculoskeletal systems.

This shift from a body designed for constant movement to one confined by prolonged sitting sets the stage for a cascade of changes. The spine remains flexed, reducing vertebral mobility. Discs lose water and become more sensitive to pressure.[3] In practice, this often shows up as stiffness when standing up after sitting, a dull ache across the lower back by the end of the workday, or the familiar "compressed" feeling many people describe before they even start moving.

As a physiotherapist, I see this most clearly in how quickly symptoms change once someone stands, walks, or gently extends their spine. Deep stabilizing muscles become less active, while superficial muscles compensate, often inefficiently. Over time, some tissues become overworked to compensate for limited movement elsewhere. However, these effects can often be improved with a few simple movements throughout the day or at least 30 minutes of daily activity.

Many people are told that sitting for 8 to 10 hours a day will shorten their hip flexors. However, true structural shortening of soft tissue typically requires prolonged immobilization rather than routine daily sitting. [4] It's important to understand that the soft tissue changes do not occur as quickly as often assumed. What people usually experience instead is stiffness driven by fatigue, protective muscle guarding, or heightened sensitivity. This is why hips may feel rigid when first standing, yet loosen noticeably within a few minutes of walking, stretching, or climbing stairs, something I see consistently across clinical settings and movement practices.

Therefore, neurological effects can play an important role in well-being. Movement provides the brain with continuous sensory information about body position, pressure, tension, and change. When movement becomes limited, the variety of sensory and motor input may also decrease.[5] In this state, the body remains present, but the brain's representation of it becomes less accurate. Prolonged screen use can worsen this effect by encouraging forward head posture, sustained neck muscle activity, and shallow breathing. Focusing the eyes on a nearby object increases nervous system activity. Many people feel stiffness, mental fatigue, or irritability after long periods of computer use. These symptoms are connected, as a protective, compressed posture keeps the nervous system on high alert.

In light of these observations, it becomes crucial to understand the implications of limited movement on our overall health. Limited range of motion is a common but often overlooked cause of pain sensitivity. Pain usually results from the nervous system's perception of threat, not from damage alone.[6] When the brain gets the same limited signals repeatedly, it becomes less confident about what the body can safely do.

This connection highlights the importance of maintaining a healthy range of motion, as it directly influences our pain perception and overall physical well-being. The spine supports a wide range of movements, such as bending, stretching, twisting, and lateral flexion, which help distribute mechanical loads. When movement is limited, stress builds up in specific areas. The nervous system then increases protective muscle tone, further restricting movement and extending the cycle. This view suggests that pain often results from prolonged periods of limited, repetitive physical activity rather than from structural abnormalities.

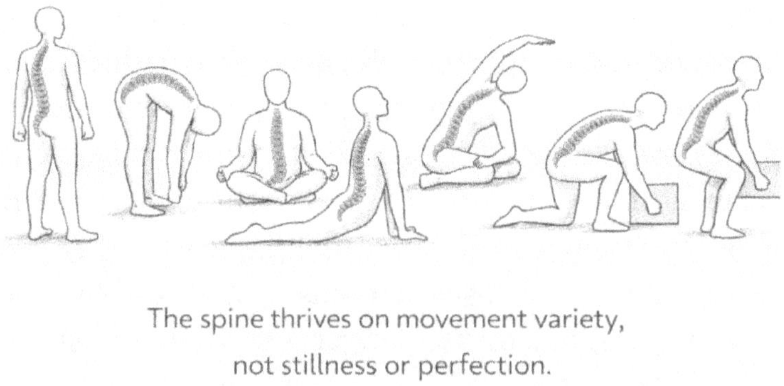

Figure 2.1: Spine movement and flexibility through poses

The Lost Art of Feeling Your Body (Somatic Disconnection)

Somatic awareness is the ability to notice what's happening inside your body, where you're holding tension, how you're positioned, the subtle sense of pressure or movement you might usually ignore. [7] This awareness is shaped by experience, but it diminishes when movement is restricted. When sitting for long periods, sensory feedback decreases: muscles and joints that remain still send fewer signals, and the brain gradually shifts its attention away from those areas. The result is a muted sense of the body, which explains why someone might rise from a chair to find one leg dull or "asleep," or why the lower back feels vague and hard to pinpoint after hours at a desk. In the clinic, people often struggle to describe what they're feeling at first, not because nothing is happening, but because the signals have been quiet for so long.[8]

Experience helps develop this awareness. In yoga classes, I often notice students lying down and realizing how uneven they feel on the mat. They might feel more weight on one shoulder, have trouble sensing one side of the pelvis, or notice tension only when things slow down. When we move less, the brain stops focusing on detailed input from these areas.

Climbing shows this even more clearly. A person might be strong enough to stand on a foothold but hesitate because they cannot feel where their weight is going. When sensory awareness returns through movement, loading, and variation, confidence often comes back right away. This is a normal physical response, not a sign of weak willpower.

Just as limited sensory awareness can undermine confidence in movement, pain adds another layer of complexity. It doesn't simply signal discomfort; it reshapes attention itself, often pulling focus away from the very area that needs it most. As a way to protect yourself, you shift your attention away.[9] While this may offer short-term relief, it typically increases disconnecting. The brain gets even less accurate information, which makes things more uncertain and, strangely, makes that area even more sensitive. This isn't a conscious choice. It's an automatic act of self-protection.

Distinguishing between pain and protective tension is essential. Pain is the brain signaling a perceived threat, while protective tension is the body's attempt to prevent harm, often before pain ever appears.[10] Many individuals experience tension before pain, yet often remain unaware until symptoms intensify due to a lack of bodily awareness. Restoring awareness involves noticing subtle bodily changes without interpreting them as threats. Research indicates that attending to bodily sensations in a gentle, nonjudgmental manner can reduce pain by calming the nervous system and improving the ability to differentiate between sensations.[11]

Individuals frequently report, "I didn't know how tense I was until I slowed down." This observation highlights how increased awareness reveals previously unnoticed patterns. Moreover, contemporary societal norms often encourage individuals to disregard bodily signals such as hunger, fatigue, and stress in pursuit of productivity. Over time, this practice creates a disconnect between bodily sensations and cognitive awareness. Addressing this disconnect is essential for effective healing.

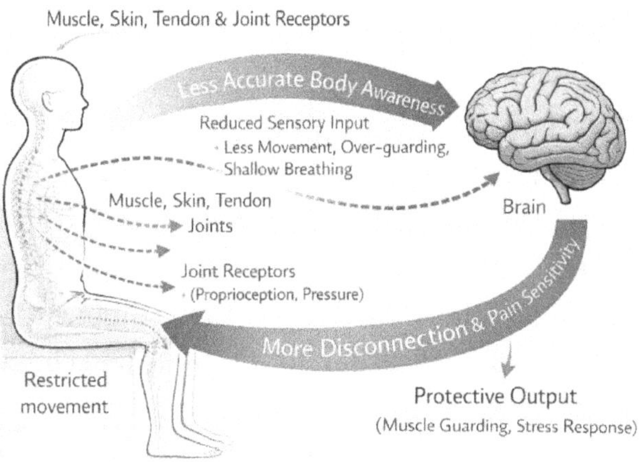

Figure 2.2: Sensory feedback loop between body and brain

Mapping Your Body's Stress Zones

Certain areas of the body are more likely to hold stress, particularly during prolonged sitting or periods of high pressure. People often notice pain in these areas because they help protect and stabilize us. The neck and jaw can get tense from staying alert, talking, or holding back emotions. The rib cage and diaphragm are linked to how we breathe and manage our feelings. The hips and lower back help keep us steady and may tense up when we feel unsafe. Stress often stays in our muscles as patterns of tension, even if we are not aware of it.[12] These patterns can start to change as we become more aware of them.

The first step in releasing tension is becoming aware of it. Many patterns of tension exist without our conscious awareness, influencing how we move, breathe, and feel. The guided scan below will help you gently notice these patterns and start connecting more deeply with your body. You don't need to fix or change your body. This scan is just a way to start listening.

Guided Tension-Mapping Scan (3 To 8 Minutes)

Begin in a comfortable seated or lying position, ensuring your body is relaxed and stable. Focus on your breath for a few cycles. Then, slowly scan your body from head to toe, starting with the jaw and face. Notice whether your teeth are gently resting or clenched, whether your tongue feels heavy or tight, and how the muscles around your eyes respond as you bring your attention there. There is no need to change anything at this stage. Shift your attention to your neck and shoulders. Observe any heaviness, tightness, or pain, noticing how it feels rather than why it's there.

Begin by focusing on your rib cage and chest. Pay attention to how your breath moves through these areas and identify any regions that may hold more tension than others. Next, shift your awareness to your lower back and hips. Take note of the sensation of the surface beneath you and any areas that may feel stiff or sore.

Continue this process by observing any sensations in your legs and feet. Remember, this scan is not for diagnosis but rather a way to identify areas of tension or stress within your body. The goal is to help your brain develop a clearer and more detailed understanding of your physical state. By repeating this practice regularly, you can gradually reduce baseline tension and cultivate greater comfort and connection within your body.

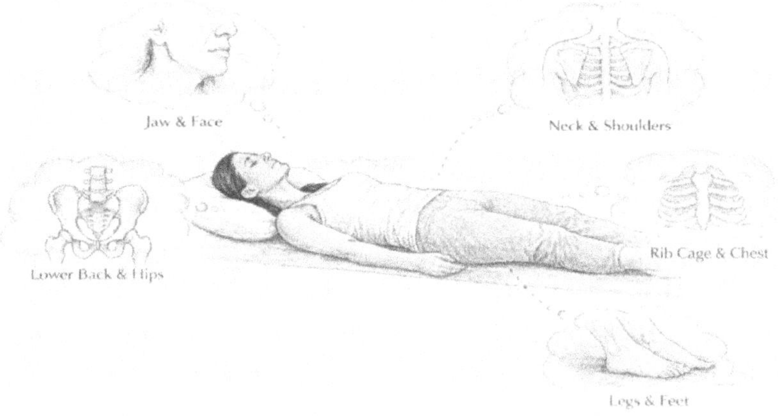

Figure 2.3: Guided Tension-Mapping Scan

Restoring Movement Confidence (Reverse Fear-Based Guarding)

Fear of moving is one of the main signs that someone might have long-term pain.[13] When the nervous system connects movement with danger, it responds by tightening muscles, reducing how much you can move, and making sensations stronger. This reaction is called guarding.[14] At first, guarding helps protect you, but over time, it can actually cause ongoing pain. Guarding is not always obvious. Often, it shows up in small habits, like holding your breath when you bend forward, tightening your jaw when you turn your head, bracing your stomach before standing up, or moving your back stiffly instead of letting each part move on its own. These habits are learned responses, often shaped by past pain, stress, or uncertainty.

However, it becomes a problem because your nervous system stops getting clear messages that movement is actually safe. Your brain receives fewer signals that movement is safe when you move less. You might feel more uncertain as the nervous system becomes even more protective over time. Pain frequently results from not being accustomed to movement rather than from movement being risky.[15]

Therefore, it's crucial to start moving slowly and safely, in ways that feel comfortable, to gain confidence and improve your movement. The objective is to teach your nervous system that movement is safe, not to overcome pain or demonstrate your strength.[16] For micro-movements in particular, this is crucial. Your brain can detect sensations with small, gentle movements that don't cause discomfort.

Moreover, taking things slowly and carefully can help you rebuild trust between your brain and body. It's helpful to notice the difference between safe discomfort and unsafe pain. Safe discomfort might feel like mild stiffness, warmth, or a gentle stretch that goes away with rest or after repeating the movement. Unsafe pain, on the other hand, often feels sharp, frightening, or gets worse, and it may make you hold your breath or feel like you need to stop right away.

With practice, you can learn to tell them apart. The exercises below are here to help you feel more confident in your movements by gently waking up your neuromuscular pathways without causing stress. Move slowly, stay within a comfortable range, and remember to breathe calmly.

Now that we've laid the groundwork for understanding your body's movements, let's focus on specific exercises to enhance your upper back mobility.

Thoracic Rotations and Chest Opening

If you spend a lot of time sitting, your upper back can become stiff. Sitting for a long time reduces rotational movement in this region, forcing the neck and lower back to compensate. Improving movement in your upper back can help reduce strain elsewhere.

Sit with your feet flat on the floor. Place one hand across your chest and the other behind your head or on your shoulder. Take a slow breath in. As you breathe out, gently turn your upper body a little to the side of the hand behind your head. Try to move from your rib cage, not your arms.

Pause for a moment, then return to the center. Repeat the movement on the other side. Keep the motion small and controlled, and stop if you feel any pain. Move slowly and let your breath guide you. Continue for one to two minutes, switching sides each time. This gentle rotation is a simple way to reassure your nervous system that your spine can move without danger.

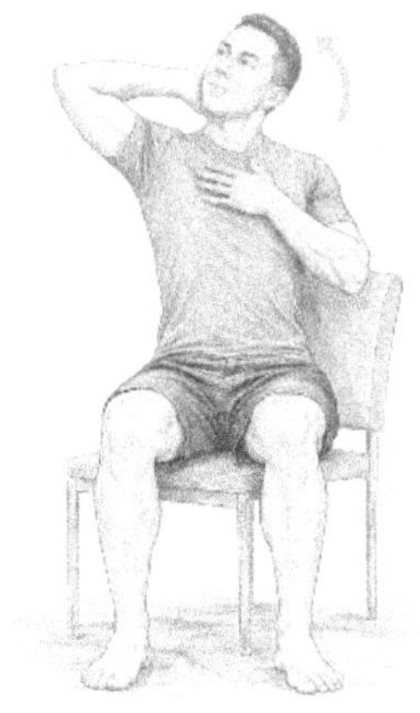

Figure 2.4: Seated thoracic rotation with neutral spine

Pelvic Tilts

If you've had pain for a while, you probably experience stiffness in the pelvis and lower back. Pelvic tilts restore gentle movement and promote mobility in both areas.

To begin this exercise, lie flat on your back with your knees bent and your feet resting flat on the floor. Place your arms comfortably at your sides. As you inhale, gently tilt your pelvis forward to create a small arch in your lower back, known as an anterior pelvic tilt. Then, as you exhale, tilt your pelvis back to relax your lower back toward the floor, which is called a posterior pelvic tilt. Move slowly and focus on the sensations in your body rather than the range of motion. Continue this movement for one to two minutes, maintaining a steady breathing pattern. This exercise can help reduce the fear of spinal movement and enhance your brain's awareness of your lower back.

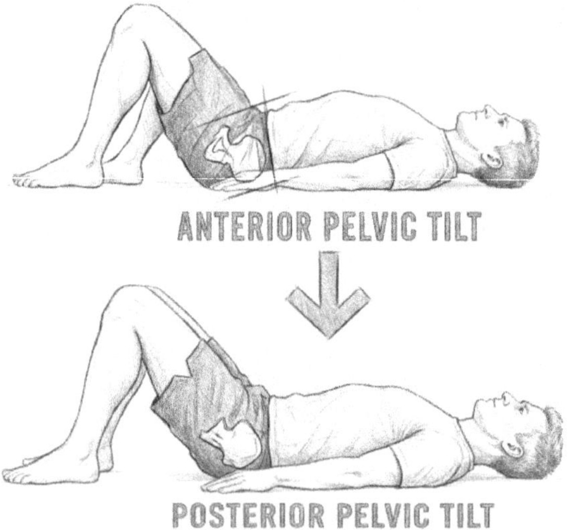

Figure 2.5: Supine pelvic tilt sequence

Neck Nods

Neck nods target the deep cervical muscles, which can become stiff when the neck remains immobile. Therefore, this exercise promotes movement without placing excessive strain on your body.

To perform this exercise, either lie on your back or sit upright with support. Gently nod your head as if saying "yes," bringing your chin slightly toward your throat, and then release. The movement should be minimal and nearly imperceptible. Move slowly, avoiding any forced stretch or tension. If you choose to lie on your back, tuck your chin and slightly lift the back of your head. When done correctly, you should feel a gentle engagement in the deep muscles at the front of your neck without any strain. Continue this for one minute, keeping your breathing relaxed, and your eyes closed. This exercise helps relax overactive muscles at the back of the neck and improves coordination of the deeper stabilizers.

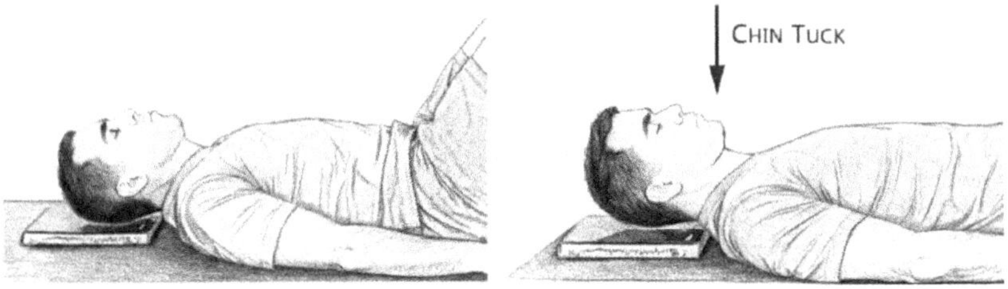

Figure 2.6: Small-range neck nod demonstration

Scapular Glides

If you're looking for a way to relieve tension in your shoulders and improve overall mobility, this mindful shoulder exercise can be a great addition to your routine.

Begin by sitting or standing comfortably with your arms relaxed. Slowly move your shoulder blades forward and backward along your rib cage, avoiding lifting or shrugging your shoulders. Next, move your shoulders in small circles, focusing on the sensation rather than the range of motion. Keep your neck relaxed throughout the exercise. Continue for one to two minutes while breathing steadily.

This exercise is especially beneficial for individuals who tend to hold tension in their shoulders, often without realizing it. Signs of tension can include keeping the shoulders slightly raised, tensed, or pulled back throughout the day. In my clinical experience, I often observe this in people who spend long hours at desks, engage in repetitive movements, experience stress, or are recovering from injuries. This exercise supports normal shoulder movement and helps relieve tension in the neck and upper back.

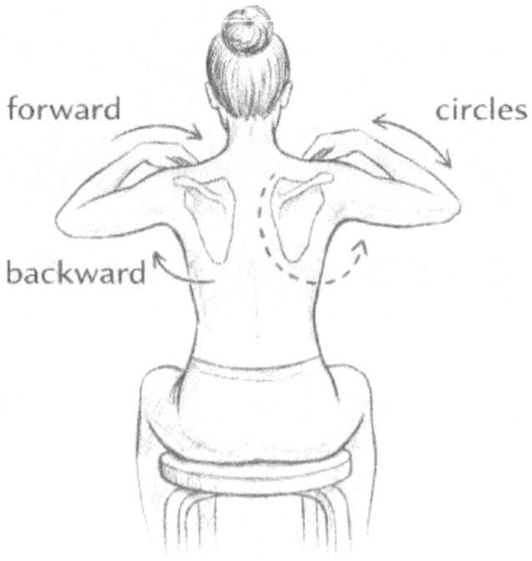

Figure 2.7: Scapular glides

Why Confidence Matters More Than Range

Right now, focusing on how well you move matters more than how far you can go. When you move with confidence, your nervous system feels safe. This helps your brain adjust and makes movement easier. As fear decreases, your range and strength will grow over time. If you try to push your range too quickly, your body may tense up, slowing your progress. Therefore, by exercising patience in your approach now, you lay the groundwork for greater improvements in the future. Embracing a gradual process allows your body to adapt and grow stronger, ultimately leading to more effective and sustainable results.

Your Action Plan

Reconnection does not happen in just one practice session. It develops through short, repeated moments of paying attention to your body during the day. The aim is not to avoid sitting completely, but to break it up with movement and awareness so your nervous system stays active.

Moreover, small movements, repeated often, are more effective for nervous system regulation than a single long workout followed by hours of stillness. If it helps to see how this might fit into a real day, here's one gentle way to spread these movements across morning, midday, and evening.

Time of Day	Focus	Activities
Morning	Start the day with breathing and gentle movement	• 2 minutes of rib mobility breathing • 2 minutes of gentle hip opening or pelvic tilts • 2 minutes of neck nods or cat-cow movement
Midday	Break up long periods of sitting with light movement	• 1 minute of chest stretches • One micro-movement for the spine (thoracic rotations, scapular glides, or neck rotations) • Ankle circles and pumps (especially if sitting most of the day)
Evening	Relax the body and release built-up tension	• 5–10 minutes of floor-based movement or gentle release • Slow breathing with awareness of ribs, hips, or neck • Cat-cow movements

Movement Snacks: Small Actions, Big Impact

Movement snacks are short bursts of light exercise you can do every 45 to 90 minutes. You do not need special clothes or equipment, and you can do them almost anywhere. For example, stand up and twist your spine, shift your weight from one foot to the other, move your shoulders, or take a few slow, deep breaths to expand your ribs. These small breaks help prevent stiffness, boost circulation, and keep your nervous system engaged.

In addition to these movement snacks, incorporating specific techniques can enhance overall mobility and relaxation.

Rib Mobility Resets

Place your hands on your rib cage and slowly take three to five breaths a few times each day. Focus on making your ribs expand out and lengthen, rather than lifting your chest. This can be especially helpful if you notice shallow breathing, chest tightness, or a sense of holding your breath during the day.

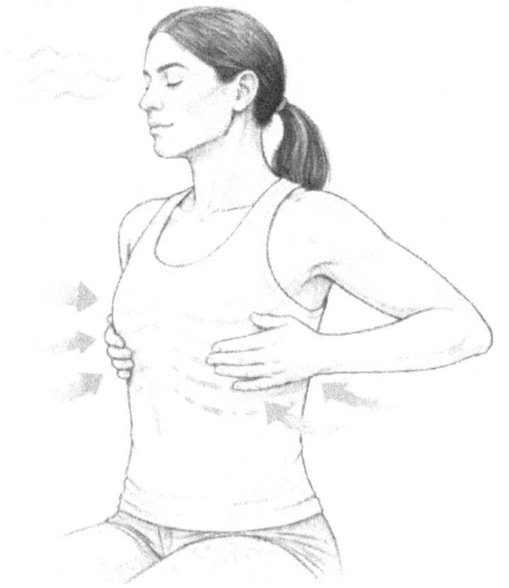

Figure 2.8: Rib mobility resets

Hip Opening Micro-Breaks

If you've been sitting for a while, stand up and step into a small lunge. Let your hips move naturally, noticing how your weight shifts through your feet and the front of the hip softens as you move. Shift gently back and forth for 30 to 60 seconds. This movement helps restore hip extension and can reduce pressure on your lower back.

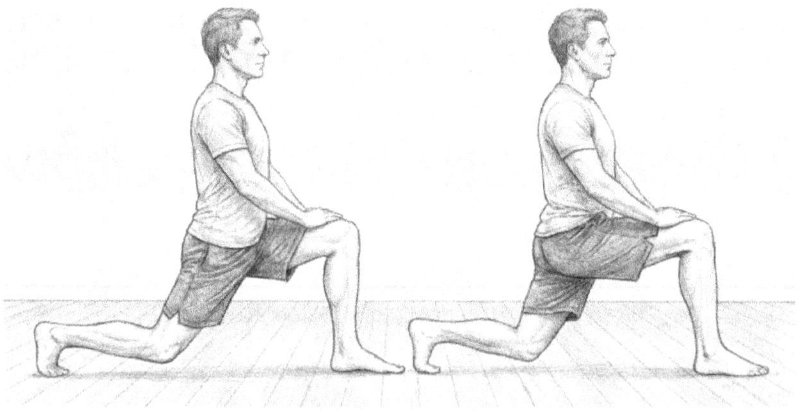

Figure 2.9: Hip opening micro-breaks

Chest Stretches

Sitting for a long time or working with your arms in front of you can make your chest muscles feel tight. Doing a quick chest stretch can help loosen them up. Stand with your feet shoulder-width apart. Find a sturdy wall or door, and reach one arm out at shoulder height, pressing your forearm and palm flat against the surface. Gently turn your body away from your arm to stretch your chest. Hold the stretch for 30 to 60 seconds, then switch sides. Notice how your breathing changes as the stretch eases, especially across the front of your ribs.

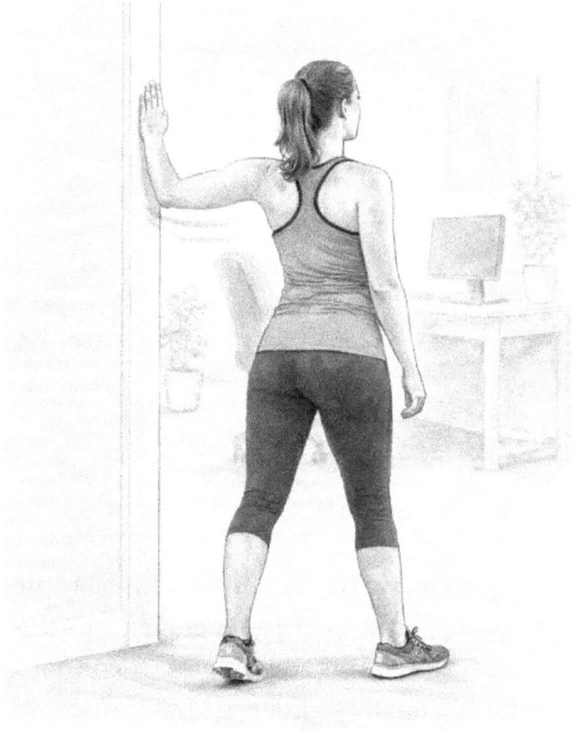

Figure 2.10: Chest stretches

Cat-Cow Movement (Gentle Spinal Reset)

This slower Cat-cow variation helps bring movement back to your spine and ribs without forcing a stretch. Rather than pushing into large shapes, focus on noticing how your spine responds to your breath and small shifts in position. Move slowly, rounding and gently arching your spine, letting your breath guide the movement rather than using force. Let your head and pelvis follow naturally. The aim is not to increase flexibility, but to reconnect with your body and remind your nervous system that your spine can move safely and smoothly. This is especially useful after sitting for a long time, when your back feels stiff or tense. Just a few slow repetitions can help release tension and make breathing easier.

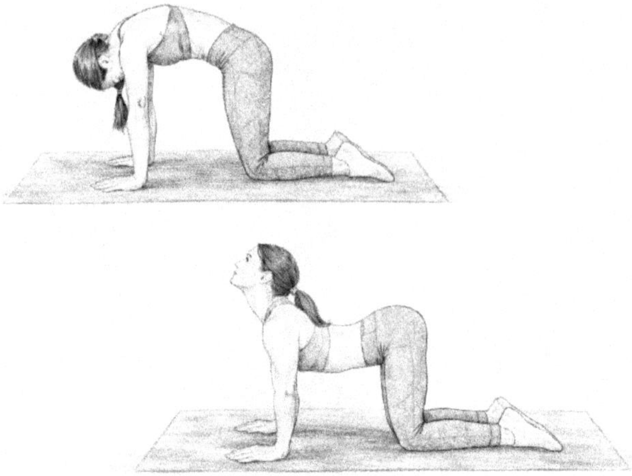

Figure 2.11: Cat-cow movement

Before moving forward, it is important to remember that these practices are not meant to be perfect routines or strict rules. They are simply tools to help you reconnect with your body throughout the day. Even a few small moments of awareness can begin to shift how your body feels and responds. Over time, these small changes build trust between your mind and body, creating the foundation for greater and more lasting improvements.

Final Thoughts

Reconnection helps calm your nervous system and restore your inner balance. If you move without awareness, your actions can feel automatic and tense. With awareness, your movements become safer and more flexible. By learning to feel your body clearly, you help your nervous system feel less uncertain. When protection softens, pain loses its grip. In the next chapter, we will focus on chronic muscle tension and explore how to release it gently, without forcing or overstretching. This is how awareness leads to real change.

CHAPTER 3

Release

When someone has chronic pain, it often reflects an overprotective nervous system rather than just weakness or tightness.

Believing your body is broken or fundamentally flawed because of chronic pain can be especially harmful. This mindset often develops gradually through repeated flare-ups, inconclusive scans, and short-lived treatments. As time goes on, pain can feel like a sign of failure, prompting you to either confront it, disregard it, or just tolerate it. This confrontation often manifests as bracing yourself, pushing through workouts, holding your breath, or mentally wrestling with discomfort.

In fact, most chronic pain does not indicate bodily failure.[1] Instead, it shows the body has been protecting itself for too long. Muscles tighten to stabilize and guard vulnerable areas, which is helpful in the short term. However, prolonged tension restricts movement, alters breathing, increases fatigue, and heightens sensitivity in the nervous system. Breathing often becomes shallow without conscious awareness. Ultimately, pain results from protective mechanisms that have outlived their usefulness, not from dysfunction.[2]

Taking this into account, this chapter emphasizes the concept of release, encouraging the body to recognize that it no longer needs to hold on so tightly. In the following section, you'll start exploring simple, body-centered practices designed to gently ease tension and rebuild trust in movement.

The Three Tension Hotspots: Neck, Ribs, Hips

Chronic stress can lead to tension in various parts of the body, but it most commonly affects the neck, rib cage, and hips. These areas are interconnected both mechanically and neurologically, working together to influence how the body responds to stress, often without our awareness. The neck plays a crucial role in orienting the head, eyes, and senses. In response to perceived threats, it can stiffen as a protective mechanism for vital areas. This chronic tension in the neck often results from prolonged screen time, sustained mental focus, and heightened emotional awareness.[3] Over time, this tension can restrict movement, cause headaches, and add stress to the shoulders and upper back.

The rib cage is vital for effective breathing, yet under stress, our breathing often becomes shallow and limited, typically relying on the upper chest. This reduces diaphragm function and rib movement, which can have significant effects on the nervous system. Restricted rib motion can maintain a heightened state of alertness, making relaxation more difficult.[4]

Similarly, the hips and pelvis serve as the body's foundation, crucial for stabilizing posture and facilitating the transfer of force between the upper and lower body. When under stress, the hips tend to tighten to ensure stability. Prolonged sitting can exacerbate this tightening, leading to stiffness, limited hip extension, and increased stress on the lower back.

Interestingly, these three areas constantly influence one another. A stiff rib cage increases strain on the neck, while restricted hips force the lower back to compensate. Neck tension alters breathing patterns, further stiffening the ribs. This interdependence explains why pain often shifts or appears in multiple areas over time.

Therefore, understanding these common stress points encourages a broader perspective, shifting the focus from isolated pain to overall movement patterns. Instead of asking, "Where does it hurt?" it can be more helpful to ask, "Where is my body staying tense or avoiding movement?"

When we look at the body this way, pain often makes more sense. For example, someone with neck pain may notice limited rib cage movement during breathing or persistent hip stiffness. In this case, the neck may be working harder to compensate for other restricted areas, rather than being weak or injured in its own right.

Because these regions are closely connected through the nervous system, they can also respond quickly when given the right kind of input. Slow breathing, gentle movement, and supported positions often create noticeable changes within minutes. This happens as the nervous system receives signals of safety and begins to reduce protective tension.[5] As this tension decreases, the body frequently feels lighter, freer, and easier to move.

Stretching Vs. Mobility Vs. Release Techniques

When people feel stiff, tight, or in pain, they often turn to stretching as the first line of defense. While stretching can be helpful, it is only one way to influence how the body moves and feels. In reality, improving movement and reducing tension usually involves three different approaches: *stretching, mobility work, and release techniques.* Although these methods may look similar from the outside, they affect the body in different ways. Understanding these differences can help you choose the most appropriate approach for your body, especially if tension or pain has been present for a long time.

Stretching: Increasing Tolerance, Not Length

Stretching is commonly used to relieve tension, though its effectiveness varies. While it reliably improves flexibility and range of motion, its precise effects on muscles and nerves remain under debate. [6] Some scientists think stretching mainly works by training your nerves to tolerate more, while others think it causes small changes in muscle structure. However, most short-term improvements in flexibility appear to result from increased stretch tolerance rather than permanent changes in muscle length.[7]

Increased flexibility may give the impression that muscles have permanently lengthened, but improvements in flexibility do not necessarily reflect lasting changes in muscle length. Instead, stretching primarily engages the nervous system, which limits muscle extension through protective mechanisms. When you stretch, muscle spindles detect changes in length and activate the stretch reflex to prevent overstretching.[8] With regular practice, the nervous system gradually allows a greater range of motion, increasing what is known as stretch tolerance.

For this reason, stretching should not be pushed into pain. In many cases, improvements in range of motion occur when the body learns to relax unnecessary muscle tension rather than forcing muscles to lengthen. Over time, consistent flexibility work can support better joint movement and coordination.[9] Stretching tends to be most effective when the nervous system feels safe and relaxed.

Mobility: Control, Coordination, and Variability

Mobility focuses on improving joint movement and control through slow, controlled motions within a comfortable range. These exercises restore coordination among joints, muscles, and the nervous system by actively engaging neural pathways, unlike passive stretching. Mobility training increases movement options and variability, thereby reducing strain from repetitive or rigid patterns.[10]

This is particularly valuable after extended periods of sitting, guarding, or avoiding movement. However, mobility alone may not be sufficient. If the nervous system still perceives a threat due to pain history, stress, or fatigue, even well-designed mobility exercises can feel challenging or ineffective. In such cases, the body may remain guarded despite good movement quality, necessitating the use of release techniques.

Release Techniques: Reducing Protection

When someone has chronic pain or stress-related tension, their muscles are usually not short, but overactive. The main issue is too much protection from the nervous system, not just weakness or tightness. Thus, release techniques help reduce muscle tone by stimulating sensory receptors that signal the nervous system that it is safe to relax. Examples include slow, supported movements, gentle pressure, oscillations, and breathing-led movements.

In this regard, studies in pain science and physiotherapy show that gentle sensory input, like slow movement, light pressure, oscillations, and breathing-led motion, can lower muscle tone by calming the nervous system.[11] This works by stimulating certain sensory pathways that help control the body's automatic responses.

Common release techniques include:

- Slow, supported movements
- Gentle pressure using hands, bolsters, or props
- Small oscillatory or rocking motions
- Movements guided by breathing rather than force

These methods do not mechanically break up tissue or release fascia. Their effects are neurological, changing how the brain interprets sensations and threats.[12] This explains why stretching provides only temporary relief. If the nervous system remains protective, tension will return after the stretch.[13]

How to Know If a Technique Is Helping

A straightforward way to assess your experiences is to observe how your body responds. Helpful techniques often lead to feelings of relaxation, warmth, openness, and slower breathing. In contrast, unhelpful techniques typically result in increased strain, effort, breath-holding, or a sense of urgency.

Imagine you are doing a chest stretch against a wall. If the technique is helpful, you might notice your shoulders gradually softening, your chest feeling more open, and your breathing becoming slower and deeper. The stretch feels comfortable, and your body naturally settles into it. However, if the technique is unhelpful, the opposite often happens. You may feel yourself pushing harder into the stretch, your shoulders tightening, or your breath becoming shallow or held. Instead of easing tension, the movement creates more effort and a sense that you need to force the position.

Release work should feel surprisingly easy. You often make progress when your nervous system lets go of trying to control everything. Stretching, mobility, and release techniques each play a role. For people who are sensitive or stressed, it usually helps to start with release, then move on to mobility, and add stretching if needed.

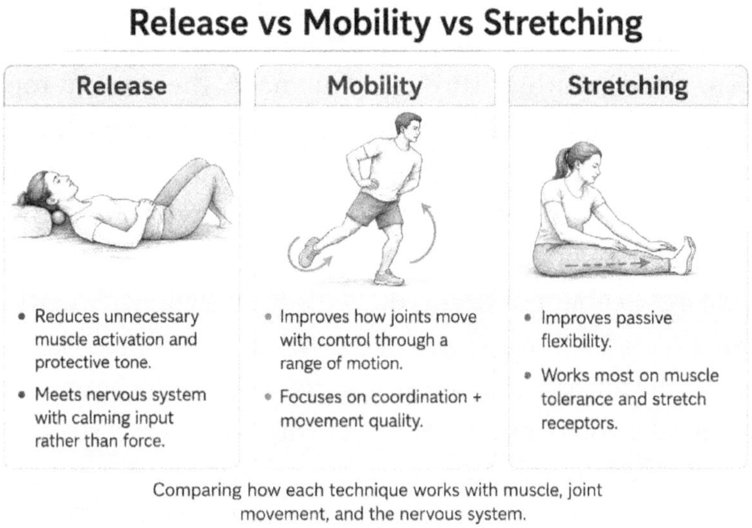

Figure 3.1: Stretching vs mobility vs release techniques comparison

Breath-Led Relaxation Techniques

Breathing is one of the most direct ways to influence your nervous system and reduce physical tension. When we feel stressed, in pain, or mentally overwhelmed, our breathing often becomes shallow, rapid, or held without us noticing. These patterns can increase muscle tension and reinforce the body's protective responses. By consciously slowing and guiding the breath, you can signal safety to your nervous system and encourage your muscles to relax. The following techniques use simple breathing patterns to reduce tension and help the body shift toward a calmer, more balanced state.

The Physiological Sigh

The physiological sigh is a natural reflex that helps lower stress and facilitates relief. To practice this relaxation technique, start by sitting or lying down comfortably. Take a deep, slow breath in through your nose, then at the top of your breath, take a second quick breath to fully expand your lungs. Slowly exhale through your mouth, allowing your chest and ribs to relax. Repeat this cycle two to four times, resting between each set.

Many people notice a reduction in tension, particularly in their neck and shoulders, as the extra air gently stretches and relaxes the muscles in those areas. This method can be especially beneficial if you're experiencing pain or high levels of stress.

Once you're familiar with the quick tension-relieving effect of the physiological sigh, you can try parasympathetic breathing to cultivate a deeper, longer-lasting calm.

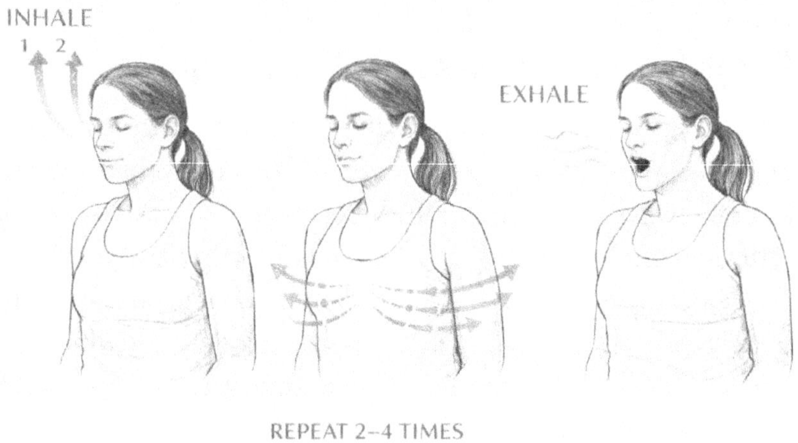

Figure 3.2: The physiological sigh

Parasympathetic Breathing

Breathing out for longer than you breathe in helps activate the parasympathetic system. One easy way to try this is to breathe in for four counts and out for six. The specific numbers are less important than finding a comfortable rhythm. Personally, I like to breathe in for four counts and out for eight. Repeat the cycle up to 8 to 10 times (around 2 minutes) or until calm. This method is most effective when you are still or moving gently.

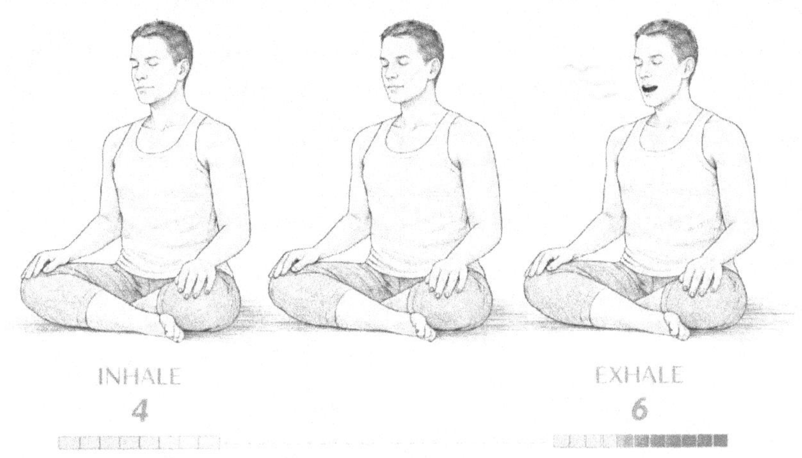

Figure 3.3: Parasympathetic breathing

Practicing these methods regularly can help you notice where tension accumulates, release it more easily, and respond to stress before it becomes chronic. Over time, breath-led relaxation becomes a tool you can carry with you throughout the day, supporting both movement and overall well-being.

Stress-Release Yoga for Pain Relief

Yoga can be a helpful way to reduce stress when practiced correctly. However, some types of yoga are not suitable for people who are in pain. Styles that use extreme stretching or require holding difficult poses can make symptoms worse by stimulating the nervous system. For stress relief, yoga should focus on support, breathing, and relaxation.[14] The poses below are recommended because they help you relax and regain confidence in movement. These are gentle poses often suggested by physiotherapists.

Supported Child's Pose (Salamba Balasana)

This pose enhances spinal flexion, hip release, and diaphragmatic breathing. Use bolsters or pillows to support the body and promote complete relaxation. Remain in the pose for 3 to 5 minutes, or as long as comfortable. Halfway through, turn your head to the opposite side. Relax your head and shoulders. Let your abdomen soften. Then gently draw your awareness inward and allow distractions to fade.

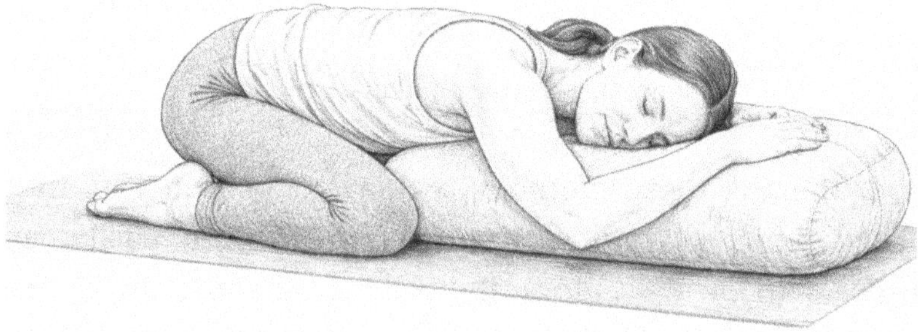

Figure 3.4: Supported child's pose

Constructive Rest (Savasana Variation with Bent Knees)

This version of Savasana is a gentle, restorative pose done lying on your back with your knees bent. It helps your hips and lower back soften, drawing your attention gently into your belly and lower spine. Practicing this pose supports diaphragmatic breathing and promotes parasympathetic activity, thereby enhancing relaxation and stress reduction.[15]

So, begin by focusing on steady breaths and let your upper body relax completely into the mat. Stay in the pose for as long as it feels good. It can be especially helpful for women with menstrual cramps or anyone with knee pain.[16] After a few minutes, you may notice deep relaxation, reduced stress, and greater mental clarity. You can also try this pose with your feet resting on a chair, which is often more comfortable than lying flat.

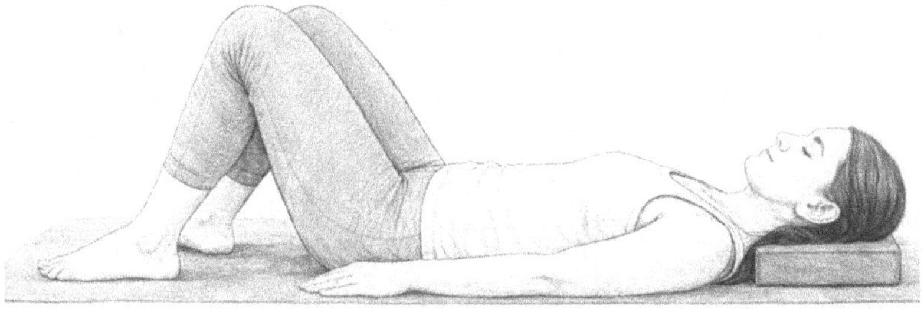

Figure 3.5: Constructive rest

Supine Twist (Supta Matsyendrasana)

To do this pose, lie on your back and cross one leg over your body. It gently stretches your spine, opens your chest, and helps release tension in your hips and lower back. You do not need to force your knee down. Just let the weight of your leg and gravity do the work. If the stretch feels too strong, try putting a pillow or block under your knee for more comfort.

Stay in the pose for 30 to 90 seconds on each side, or up to 2 minutes if it feels good, and your breathing is easy. Switch sides slowly and rest on your back for a moment between twists. Try to keep your breathing slow and relaxed. If you notice you are holding your breath or feel any discomfort, ease out of the pose or make the twist smaller. Focus on letting go, not on how far you can twist.

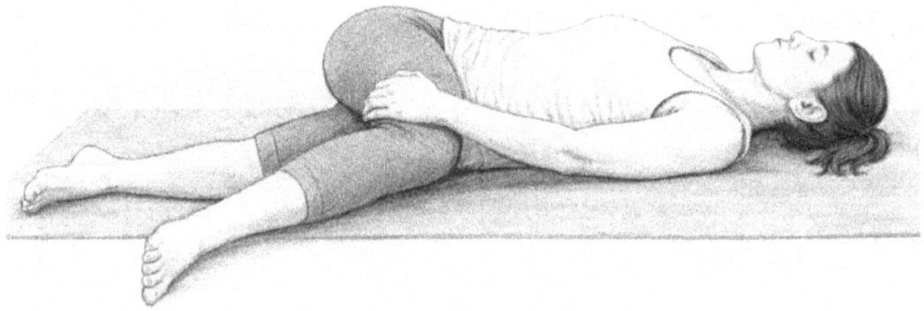

Figure 3.6: Supine twist

Seated Forward Fold (Paschimottanasana)

Paschimottanasana is a classic yoga pose that deeply stretches the back body, from the calves and hamstrings to the spine. While it might look like a simple fold, this posture goes far beyond flexibility, encouraging patience, introspection, and breath awareness.

For many people, this pose elicits immediate resistance: tight hamstrings, a pulling sensation along the back of the legs, lower back strain, or a sense of frustration when the body doesn't move the way they expect it to.

If you feel stuck or discouraged here, that's completely normal. This posture often reveals where the body is still protecting itself. Using support and limiting your range of motion allows you to release tension safely without overstretching. You are free to adjust or exit the pose at any time.

When practiced mindfully, this forward fold calms the nervous system and may support digestive comfort through relaxation and diaphragmatic breathing.[17] It is commonly used in Hatha, Vinyasa, Yin, and Restorative classes to create space in both body and mind. Rather than pushing into discomfort, focus on safety and awareness to relieve pain.

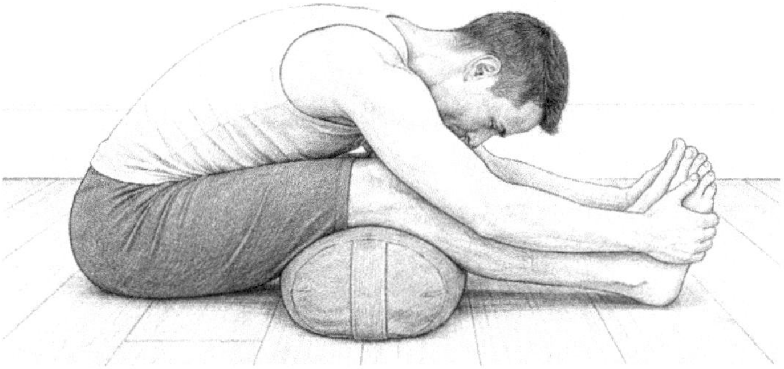

Figure 3.7: Seated forward fold

Downward-Facing Dog (Adho Mukha Svanasana)

Downward-facing dog is a full-body pose that lets your spine, shoulders, hips, and ribs move together while staying within a comfortable range. Distributing the load across multiple joints may feel more supportive than isolated stretching, particularly for individuals with pain sensitivity. Bending the knees frequently increases pelvic mobility, reduces strain on the lower back and hamstrings, and promotes natural spinal elongation. Relaxing your head can ease neck tension and help your nervous system feel calmer.

To avoid putting too much weight on your shoulders, press gently into the floor and let your shoulder blades move smoothly along your rib cage. Focus on feeling supported, rather than sinking into your shoulders. If you feel any discomfort, try bending your knees more or come out of the pose.

This pose works well as a reset, not just a stretch. Try shifting your weight a little, gently pedaling your feet, or moving your spine slightly to boost circulation and ease stiffness without extra effort. You can hold downward dog for different lengths of time, but I suggest starting with 30 to 90 seconds, as long as your breathing stays steady. You can also add slow movement, moving between the downward dog and the plank. Exhale as you move into downward dog and inhale as you shift into plank. This helps connect your breath, strength, and control. When practiced this way, the pose often leaves you feeling lighter, more grounded, and more at ease.

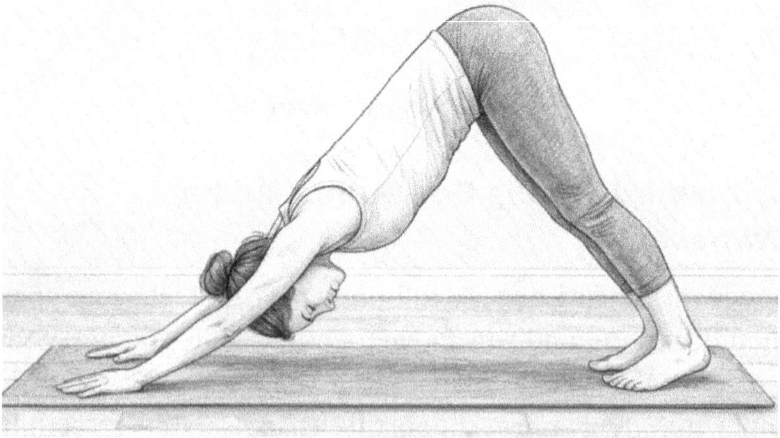

Figure 3.8: Downward-facing dog

Extended Triangle Pose (Utthita Trikonasana)

The extended triangle pose is a steady standing posture that promotes grounding through the legs while gently opening the chest and rib cage. When practiced mindfully, yoga postures like this may support stress reduction and autonomic regulation.

The Extended triangle pose teaches the body to distribute weight evenly across the legs, pelvis, spine, and rib cage rather than forcing flexibility in one area. Stability begins with the feet and legs, allowing the spine to lengthen and rotate with control. The goal is to maintain steady breathing and ease, not to reach the floor. Using a block or placing the hand higher on the leg can help reduce strain and support relaxation. Comfort matters more than form.

So, begin by holding this pose for 20 to 45 seconds per side, or practice it dynamically with small, breath-guided movements. Performed gently, it enhances balance, rib mobility, and standing confidence without increasing tension.

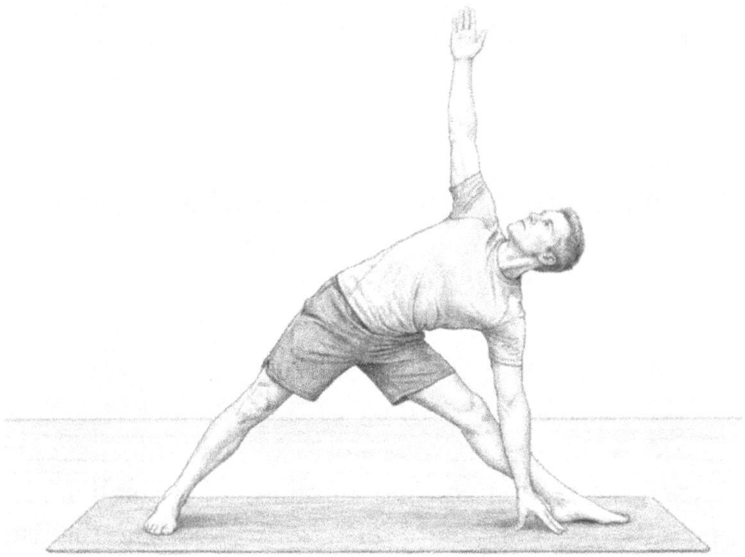

Figure 3.9: Extended Triangle Pose

Action Steps: The 5-Minute Daily Release Flow

Flow Release does not require lengthy sessions, strict routines, or ideal conditions. Consistency and awareness of the nervous system's responses are key. When practiced as a daily routine rather than as a problem-solving tool, its benefits accumulate over time. The five-minute release flow targets tension in the neck, ribs, and hips, areas that often tighten without us noticing during long days of sitting, stress, or mental overload, and promotes safety by emphasizing breath and attention.

You can practice it once or twice daily, or as needed during periods of stress or discomfort. This flow is not a replacement for exercise, strength training, or rehabilitation, but it prepares the body so that other movements become easier and more effective.

Neck Release: Reducing Tension

Chronic neck tension may present as stiffness, pressure, or heaviness in the head and neck. This tension is rarely caused by weakness alone. More often, it results from sustained vigilance and prolonged low-level muscle activation associated with stress.[18]

Start by sitting or standing comfortably, ensuring your back is supported and your feet are flat on the ground. Let your shoulders rest in a natural position. Shift your focus to the sides of your neck and the base of your skull. Gently turn your head a few degrees to each side, pausing briefly at the end of each rotation before returning to the center. Remember to breathe slowly and relax your jaw throughout the movement.

Once that feels easy and familiar, add small nodding movements, as if saying "yes," while keeping the range limited. Avoid pulling or stretching. Notice if your shoulders, jaw, or breath become involved. If so, slow down further. True release often occurs during moments of calm rather than effort. Continue for one to two minutes.

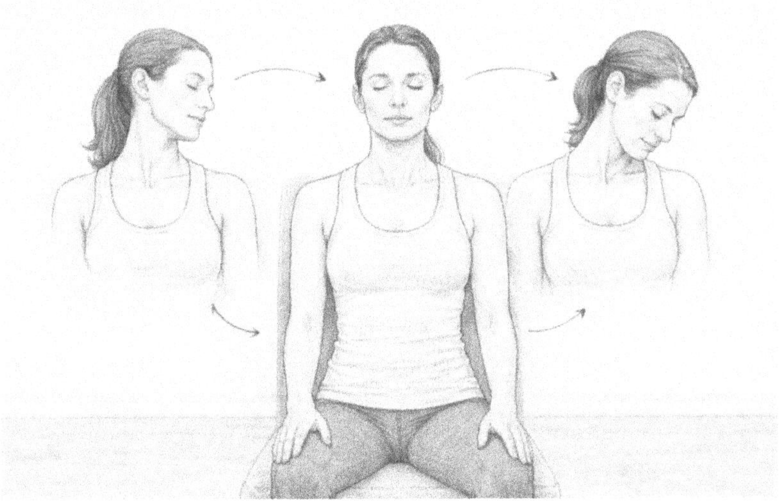

Figure 3.10: Small-range neck movements

Hip Release: Improving Mobility and Reducing Tension

Many people believe the hips store emotions, but they are also important for back health. When hips are tense or have limited movement, they can become stiff or heavy, which may lead to lower back pain. Therefore, a hip release focuses on letting go of unnecessary tension rather than forcing flexibility. Gentle movement and graded exposure may help reduce protective muscle guarding.[19]

Lie on your back with your knees bent and feet flat on the floor. Let your pelvis relax in its natural position. Gently tilt your pelvis and rock it back and forth as you breathe, keeping the movement small and easy. Then, let your knees move gently from side to side, either together or one at a time, as long as it feels comfortable.

This helps your hips move without any strain. You can also bring one knee to your chest, then release it and switch sides. Avoid pulling or stretching. Let gravity and your breath guide you. Stay in this position for one to two minutes.

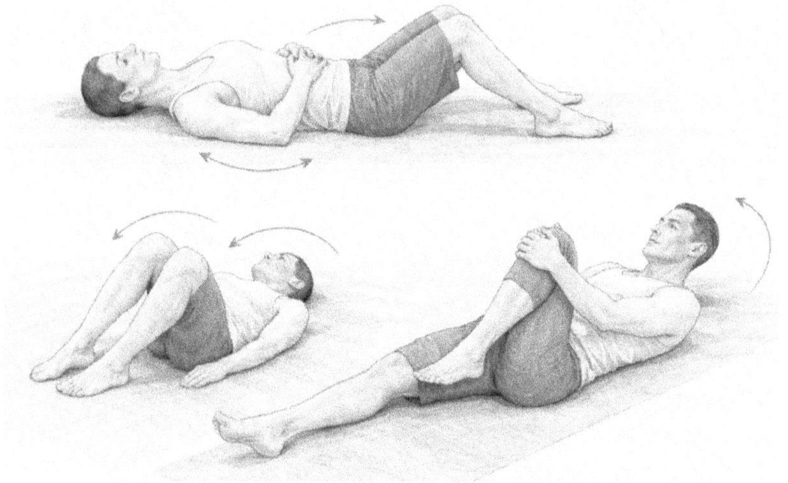

Figure 3.11: Hip and knee sequence on the floor

How to Know You're Doing It Right

The most helpful sessions often feel simple and small. When your practice is working, you might notice warmth or softness in your body, easier breathing, and a general sense of openness. At first, it's normal to notice tension more clearly. This is okay. Usually, you become aware of tension before you can let it go. Over time, your nervous system learns it doesn't have to hold on so tightly.

If you feel sharp pain, more anxiety, or a strong urge to force the movement, the practice may be too intense. Try making your movements smaller, slowing down, or just focus on breathing. Consistency matters more than how long you practice. Practicing for five minutes every day is better than doing a long session only once in a while.

Real-World Example: When Release Changes Everything

Many people notice that their pain changes after starting daily release practices. Instead of being constant or unpredictable, pain often becomes quieter, more focused, and less overwhelming.

For example, someone with chronic neck and back pain might find that, after a few weeks of daily practice, flare-ups still occur but resolve more quickly. The body stops reacting with full tension. They may find that turning their head while driving no longer triggers the same sharp tension, or that getting out of bed in the morning feels less guarded and stiff. The body stops reacting with full tension. Movements that once felt risky begin to feel lighter, even before pain has completely disappeared. Moving feels safer, and confidence grows. This shift doesn't happen because muscles suddenly get longer or stronger. It happens because the nervous system learns it doesn't need to protect the body as much.[20]

Release Is Not a Collapse

A common misunderstanding about release is that it means becoming floppy, weak, or passive. In reality, healthy release actually helps you move better. When you let go of extra tension, your body responds and works more efficiently. Release and strength go hand in hand. Strength built on a foundation of chronic tension often reinforces pain. Strength built on a foundation of relaxed muscles and awareness supports resilience. That's why release is its own important step in this process, not just something that happens at the end.

Integrating Release into Daily Life

Recognizing the significance of release, you can practice the five-minute flow on its own, but it's even more effective when you add moments of release to your daily routine. For example, try relaxing your jaw while you drive, letting your shoulders drop as you walk, or taking a deep breath into your ribs during a work break. These small pauses help your nervous system slow down. With time, release will feel less like an action and more like something that happens naturally.

Final Thoughts

By now, you may notice you handle stress differently. Instead of seeing it as an enemy, you recognize it as a signal. Tension shows your body has been working to protect you. Let it go and thank your body for its effort. This step marks the shift from just surviving to becoming more adaptable. Your body is now ready to learn how to better care for itself. Your nervous system is calmer, your awareness has returned, and chronic tension has eased.

In the next chapter, we'll look at alignment and support. This isn't about forcing perfect posture, but about finding a dynamic way to organize your body that eases strain and spreads out effort. This step helps you move from release to stability, so you can rebuild strength without pain.

CHAPTER 4

Realign

Pain doesn't come from bad posture—it comes from repeated, restricted movement.

By this step, many people have already started to change how they think about pain. They no longer see it as just a mechanical problem or a sign that something is permanently wrong. They now understand how stress, nervous system sensitivity, and chronic tension play a role. Still, one idea often sticks: the belief that pain comes from poor posture and that the answer is to find and hold the "correct" position. This makes sense because posture is easy to see, point out, and correct. It gives people something clear to focus on. In clinical practice, I often see people constantly monitoring how they sit or stand, pulling their shoulders back, tightening their core, or trying to "sit up straight" for hours at a time. But focusing solely on posture often takes people farther from lasting relief.

It's because realignment is not about fixing posture. It is about bringing back natural movement patterns so the body can support itself without extra effort. Pain usually does not come from sitting, standing, or moving "wrong" once or twice, and your body is far more resilient than you've been led to believe.[1]

Pain tends to develop when the same movement, or lack of movement, is repeated the same way again and again, without variation or rest.

For this reason, this chapter views alignment as something that changes rather than as fixed. Instead of aiming for the "perfect" shape, the goal is to help the whole body become flexible, coordinated, and easy to move.

The Myth of "Perfect Posture"

The idea of perfect posture is so common that many people never question it. You may have heard advice like sit up straight, pull your shoulders back, brace your core, or keep your head aligned with your spine. While these suggestions are usually well-meaning, they don't fully reflect how the body actually works. There is no single posture that guarantees freedom from pain. Any position, even one considered ideal, can cause discomfort if held for too long. Our bodies are designed to move and adjust rather than remain fixed in one position.[2]

You may have heard the saying, "The best posture is always the next posture." This idea captures something important: posture is meant to change. Even when you appear still, your body is constantly making small adjustments. Your weight shifts from side to side, different muscles take turns working, and your spine moves just enough to spread out the load. These small changes help prevent the same tissues from being overworked.

Problems can begin when this natural variability disappears. When discomfort shows up, many people try to control their posture very carefully, as if one wrong movement might make things worse. They stiffen their spine, tighten their stomach muscles, and move less overall. While this can feel protective at first, it often creates more strain. Holding the body rigidly reduces natural feedback, increases

muscle tension, and can keep the nervous system in a heightened state of alert.[3]

Additionally, how you feel emotionally also affects your posture. Stress, anxiety, tiredness, and feeling down can all change the way your body holds itself.[4] Some people slump, while others stiffen and sit up straight with effort. These reactions are normal and show how your body is coping. If you try to force your posture without dealing with these feelings, you might just add more tension.

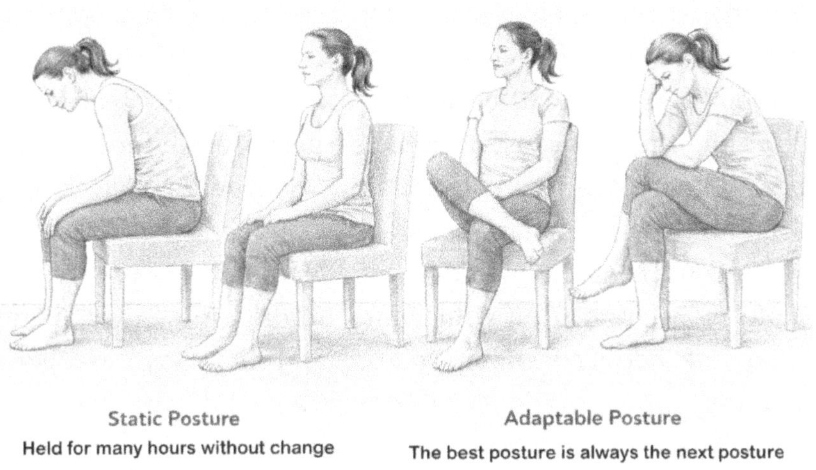

Figure 4.1: Static posture versus adaptable posture

To start improving your alignment, it's important to let go of the notion that there is only one correct way to sit or stand. The main goal is to enable your body to move easily and comfortably through various positions.

The True Meaning of Neutral Spine

Many people believe that maintaining a neutral spine means keeping it in a specific position throughout all activities. However, the truth is that neutral spine is not just a single stance; it's a range that allows your spine to effectively bear weight while still enabling you to move and breathe comfortably.

However, when individuals focus too intently on "holding neutral," they often end up bracing their bodies, causing tension in their abs and locking their ribs, which restricts their ability to breathe freely and comfortably. This makes the body stiff instead of stable. You can usually feel when your alignment is close to neutral, because the movements become smoother, your muscles work together better, and breathing feels easier.

Recent research questions the idea that there is only one "safe" way to position your spine. Studies show there is no clear link between spinal posture and pain or injury.[5] For example, athletes who often lift with a rounded back are not more likely to have back pain than those who keep their spines straight. This shifts the conversation. Therefore, instead of asking, "Is spinal flexion dangerous?" it's more useful to ask, "Can you control your range of motion?" The idea of a neutral spine is still helpful, not because it is the only safe position, but because it provides a starting point for healthy movement. From there, it's important to remember that your spine is designed to move, adapt, and handle different loads.

In fact, your spine is built to move and bend, which allows it to respond effectively to various physical demands. This inherent flexibility and strength enable your body to adapt to various stresses and activities, ensuring you maintain overall spinal health while performing daily tasks or exercising.

Problems arise when the spine flexes beyond your controllable range, particularly if the hips, thoracic spine, or core lack sufficient mobility or strength to distribute the load. This is common in individuals with limited hip rotation or tight hip capsules. When the hips cannot rotate or move effectively, the lower back compensates. Rounding your back becomes problematic because the surrounding joints are not adequately contributing, not because flexion is inherently harmful.

So, do you always need to keep your spine neutral? Sometimes you do, but not always.

In some situations, a neutral spine is beneficial, but it is not always necessary. Neutral refers to a range rather than a fixed shape. Controlled flexion is normal, and research confirms that spinal flexion is not inherently dangerous.

Training the body to move confidently through its full range of motion enhances resilience. A strong spine is not solely defined by its ability to remain straight; rather, it is characterized by its capacity to bend, flex, and rotate while maintaining stability and comfort.

To achieve this, it's essential to engage in exercises that promote awareness, control, and strength throughout the spine. One effective method is to move slowly, segment by segment, starting from the pelvis and traveling upward. This gentle exploration of flexion and extension allows you to pause briefly at the end of each range, avoiding any forcing or straining.

As you practice, remember to breathe calmly throughout the movement. The emphasis here is not on aggressive stretching but on realizing where you can move with ease and where the movement feels less smooth. This mindful approach not only improves spinal awareness but also builds confidence and strength. Current research underscores the importance of these qualities for long-term spine health, further highlighting the value of integrating such exercises into your routine.

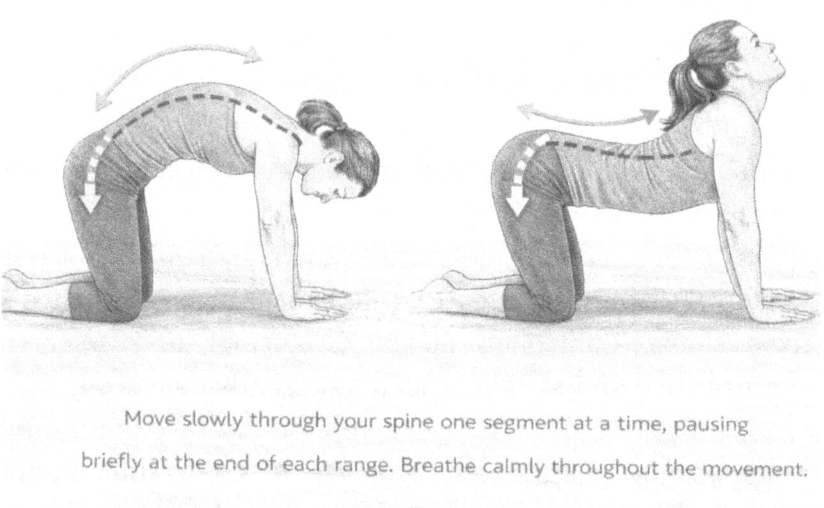

Figure 4.2: Segmental cat–cow with end-range pause

Movement Adaptability: The Real Secret to Pain-Free Living

An essential component of recovery is understanding that there is no single correct way to move. The body stays strong by adapting. Pain often shows up when movement options are restricted, not because a movement is 'wrong.' [6] When the nervous system senses only one safe way to move, it can become protective, increasing muscle tension and stiffness.

Expanding movement options improves adaptability, range of motion, and confidence, thereby reducing pain.

That's why it is important to understand that there isn't a single "best" way to lift objects—sometimes bending at the hips works best, other times using the knees distributes the load effectively. Gradually exploring different movement strategies builds physical capacity and resilience.

The same principle applies to sitting. Remaining in one posture, even if "correct," can cause strain. Changing positions, using varied supports, standing periodically, or sitting on the floor gives the body the movement it needs.

Walking illustrates this further: it involves arm swing, rib rotation, pelvic motion, and head movement. When walking becomes rigid, discomfort often follows. Therefore, reducing fear of movement is a significant predictor of improved outcomes.[7] When the neuromuscular system perceives the body as adaptable, protective muscular tension tends to decrease.[8]

I often tell my patients that staying healthy depends on moving, not avoiding movement. Being afraid to move can worsen stiffness and pain, but gradually returning to activity can help you feel more confident and reduce discomfort. Even if you have a disc herniation, degeneration, or a history of injury, movement is still important. Rest alone does not heal injured tissues. They get stronger and adapt when you gently use them in different ways.

If you avoid movement, your body becomes more sensitive, but moving again helps you build tolerance. The goal is to become adaptable, not to have perfect form. As your nervous system learns that your body can move safely in different ways, your muscles relax, and tension decreases.

When that happens, curiosity can replace fear and help you recover.

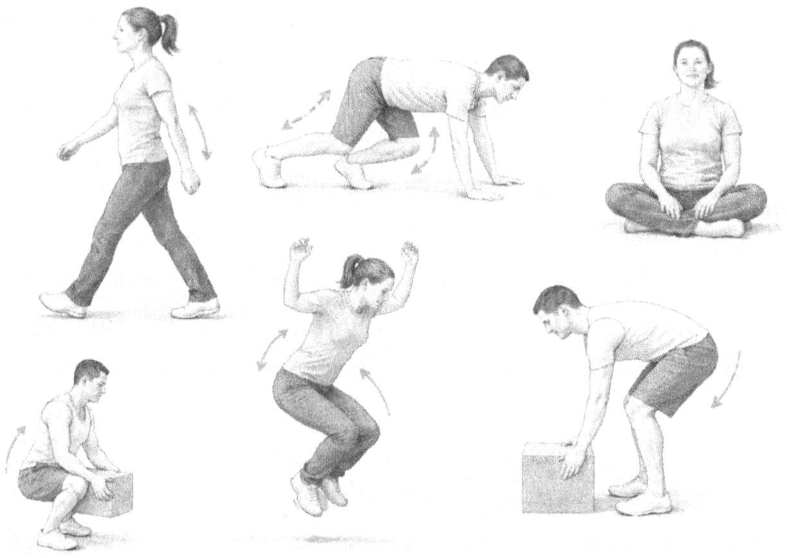

Figure 4.3: Movement adaptability

Practical Exercise

Pick a simple daily movement, like bending down to pick something up. Start by letting your hips move freely. Then, try bending your knees more. After that, incorporate a gentle movement through your spine. Use a light load and take your time with each version. Pay attention to how each variation feels. There's no need to determine which one is the best; instead, aim to provide your nervous system with a variety of options and experiences. Approach this with curiosity rather than judgment, and allow your body to guide you on what feels possible.

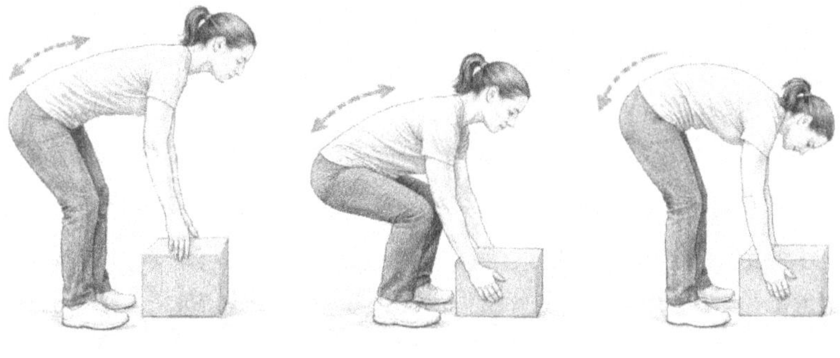

Figure 4.4: Different lifting strategies for the same task

Action Steps: The Realignment Mini-Sequence

Realignment doesn't require long sessions or complicated routines; it's about making small, repeated changes that allow your body to respond naturally. The best posture isn't just one "correct" position; it's simply the next position you move into. Using short mini-sequences helps your hips, ribs, and neck work together, making it easier to sit, stand, and move, so your posture feels more natural.

You can incorporate these sequences once or twice a day or whenever you feel stiff, tired, or mentally overloaded, especially after prolonged sitting or standing. Each movement should feel slow, controlled, and comfortable; if any movement increases pain or tension, reduce the range or slow down. On busy days, consider setting a timer for every 30 to 60 minutes to remind yourself to move. Remember, it's not about working out hard at your desk, but rather breaking up long periods of stillness. Even a minute or two of movement can help you feel refreshed and focused throughout the day.

Here are 5 simple mini-sequences to rotate throughout the day. These routines can break up periods of stillness and remind your body that it can move. Choose one or two during your breaks or try different ones as you go.

1. Shoulder and Chest Reset: Scapular Squeezes

The scapular squeeze exercise, also known as "shoulder blade squeezes," helps wake up the muscles between your shoulder blades, which often get lazy when you sit for long periods. It's a simple yet effective exercise that can help with overall shoulder health and function, as well as help you maintain a comfortable posture.[9]

Start with your elbows bent at 90 degrees. Move your forearms outwards (shoulder external rotation) while squeezing your shoulder blades together. See the picture for reference (you can also keep your elbows in touch with your ribs and just rotate forearms).

Then, relax your shoulders and return to your starting position. This exercise helps prevent rounded shoulders and reduces neck and upper-back tension caused by prolonged sitting.

Repeat 6 to 10 slow movements.

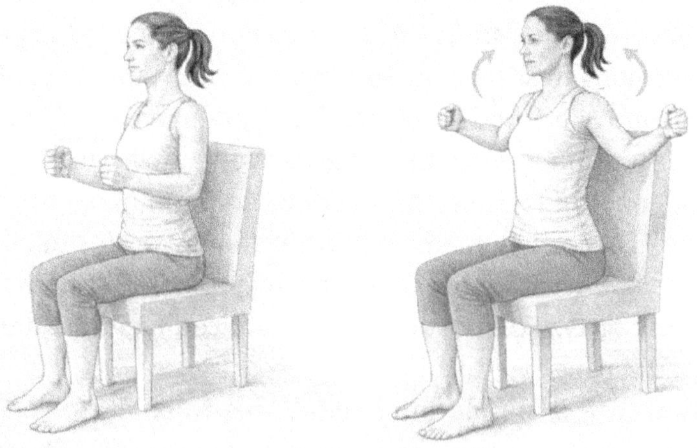

Figure 4.5: Scapular squeezes

2. Thoracic Rotation Reset: Improve Spinal Movement

Sit upright in a chair with your feet flat on the floor. Place one hand on the back of the chair or armrest and the other hand on your knee or thigh. As you exhale, gently turn your upper body to one side, focusing on moving your ribs instead of pulling with your arms. Pause for a moment, return to the center, and then turn to the other side. Keep your movements smooth and stay within a comfortable range.

This exercise helps your upper spine move better and can ease strain on your neck and lower back.

Switch sides for 30 to 60 seconds.

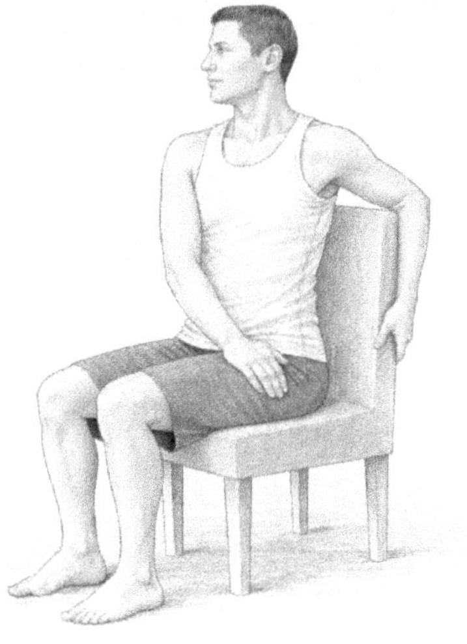

Figure 4.6: Thoracic rotations

3. Neck Reset: Releasing Muscle Tension

Place your right hand on top of your head and gently pull your head to the right. Stop when you feel a stretch on the left side of your neck. Hold for 10 to 20 seconds, then let go. Take a deep breath, then repeat on the other side, using your left hand to turn your head left until you feel a gentle stretch.

To relax the back of your neck, lower your head forward so your chin moves toward your chest. You can use your hand to gently add a bit more stretch, but do not push too hard. Hold for 10 to 20 seconds. This exercise calms overactive neck muscles and often reduces headaches and upper-body tension. This is especially helpful on days when your shoulders feel like they're creeping up toward your ears without you noticing.

Try to spend about 1 to 3 minutes on these stretches.

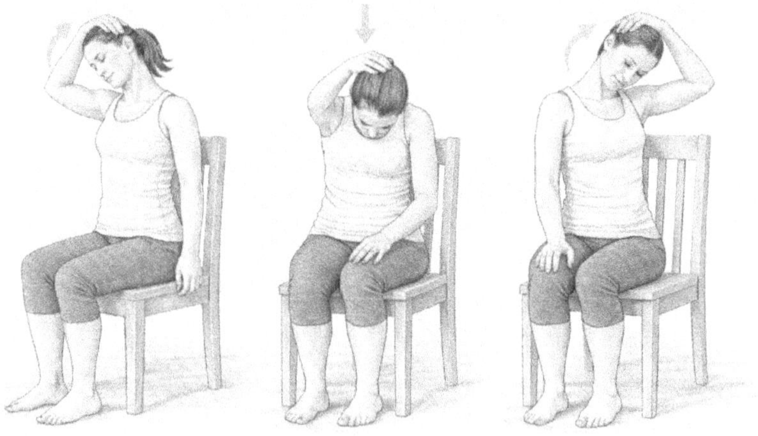

Figure 4.7: Neck pain relief stretches

4. Standing Side and Forward Bend Reset: Letting the Spine Move

Begin by standing with your feet hip-width apart. Slowly bend forward, allowing your arms to hang naturally. If necessary, bend your knees for comfort. Gently shift your weight from side to side, then gradually return to a standing position. You can also add gentle side bends, focusing on relaxing your ribcage instead of pushing the stretch. This movement helps decompress the spine and promotes fluidity after extended periods of sitting or standing.

Do this sequence for 30 to 90 seconds, and remember to breathe slowly and steadily the whole time.

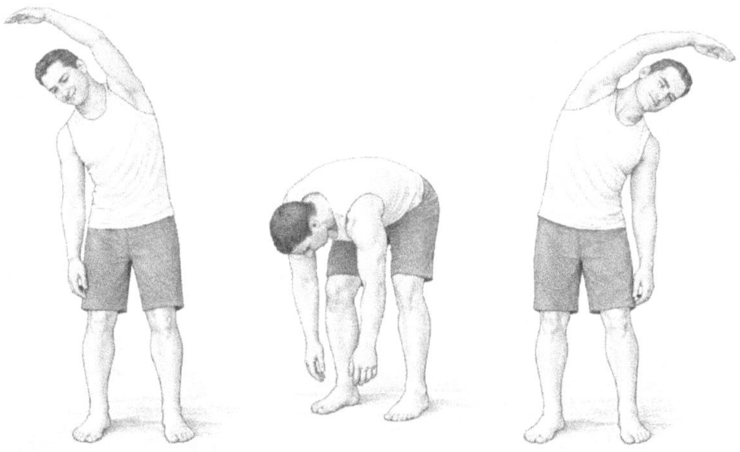

Figure 4.8: Standing spine bends

5. Seated or Standing Calf Raise Reset: Wake up Your Lower Legs

Sit or stand with your feet hip-width apart. If necessary, use a chair or desk for support to maintain balance. Lift your heels as high as you can, then pause for a moment at the top. Lower your heels back down slowly. To increase the difficulty, apply gentle pressure to your thighs with your hands to add resistance.

This exercise improves circulation, decreases lower-leg stiffness associated with prolonged sitting, and promotes better integration of foot and ankle movement with the rest of the body.

Do 10 to 20 slow reps, one to three times a day.

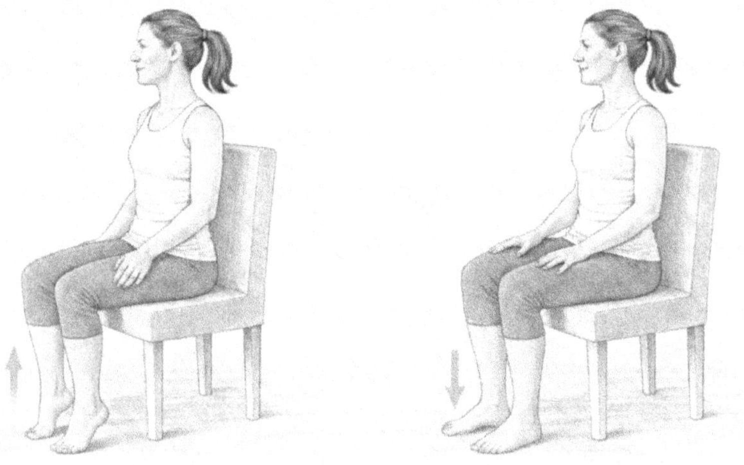

Figure 4.9: Seated calf raise

Real-World Example

Many people report that once they stop trying to maintain "perfect" posture and instead focus on a variety of movements, pain becomes more predictable and manageable. For example, someone with long-standing lower back pain may notice that changing sitting positions throughout the day reduces stiffness more than sitting upright all the time. Another person may find that allowing gentle spinal movement during lifting reduces fear and tension. These changes may seem simple, but they address the core issue: restricted movement patterns.

Over time, these small adjustments create a feedback loop: as movement variety reduces stiffness and fear, the nervous system begins to trust the body more. This trust allows for even greater freedom of motion, which not only lessens pain but also sets the stage for building strength and resilience. By practicing different ways of moving in daily life, the body learns to support itself efficiently, creating a natural transition from managing discomfort to enhancing functional capacity.

Final Thoughts

Realignment serves as the connection between release and strength. This process enables the body to maintain support without unnecessary tension and prepares it to handle physical loads confidently. The influence of pain diminishes significantly when movement patterns are diversified and well-coordinated. In the next chapter, we'll build on what you've learned by showing how to develop strength that builds confidence. Strength is most effective when your body moves easily. This step prepares you for that.

CHAPTER 5

Stabilize and Strengthen

Strength doesn't eliminate pain—it gives your body options. And options are what make you pain-resilient.

At this stage, many people notice an important change. Their pain might still be there, but it feels different. It's not as sharp or frightening, and it doesn't control their choices as much. The body feels calmer, movement is more predictable, and things don't seem as fragile anymore.

This is the moment where strength becomes useful.

People often misunderstand strength when it comes to pain. Some see it as a cure for everything, while others avoid it out of fear. Neither way is very helpful. Strength alone won't make pain disappear, and avoiding it for too long can leave your body less ready for daily life.

This step, therefore, isn't about lifting heavy weights or pushing your limits. It's about practicing strength in ways that feel steady, controlled, and repeatable, the kind that builds confidence instead of fear. It's about building a body that feels capable. A body that trusts itself under load is essential for optimal performance. This trust enables the body to absorb stress without reacting defensively, allowing for a stable foundation during workouts. Once this level of confidence and stability is achieved, you can seamlessly progress to more intense workouts and heavier lifting, as your body is prepared to handle the increased demands.

Strength and Pain: Not Always Opposites

Strength matters because life is physical. Everyday tasks like standing up, carrying groceries, reaching overhead, climbing stairs, lifting children, and getting out of the car all put stress on the body. When tissues are better prepared for that load, they tend to react with less irritation.[1] It's because stronger muscles act as shock absorbers. They distribute force more evenly across joints and connective tissue, reducing strain on passive structures. In many cases, this alone can reduce discomfort.

Strength also influences the nervous system. When movements feel stable and controlled, the system receives a clear signal that the body can handle what's being asked of it.[2] This sense of ability lowers protective tension, and less tension usually means less pain. Still, strength alone isn't always enough. This is where a lot of people get stuck. They're doing everything 'right,' exercising, getting stronger, following the plan, and yet the pain doesn't go away. That can feel confusing and discouraging. The reason is that chronic pain is rarely caused by physical load alone. It is also influenced by stress, sleep, emotions, movement habits, and fear.[3] Strength helps, but it can't fix everything if the whole system is overwhelmed.

This is why the goal isn't just to get stronger. The real goal is resilience. A resilient body recovers faster, adapts better, and responds rather than just reacts. This ability to recover and adapt is what makes a body feel dependable. And that dependability is where confidence starts. When people trust their bodies, they move more easily. The sense of freedom significantly lowers feelings of threat, which in turn can reduce sensitivity to pain. While strength plays a crucial role in this process, it is important to note that this strength must be cultivated in a manner that fosters trust rather than creates tension. By prioritizing trust, we can further enhance the sense of freedom and, in turn, mitigate pain more effectively.

Real Stability: Coordination, Timing, Breath

Stability is often confused with stiffness. Many believe being stable means tightening everything and holding on. True stability is achieved through coordination. Stable movement happens when muscles activate in the right sequence, at the right moment, and with the appropriate level of effort. Stability is dynamic and responsive rather than rigid, and breathing plays a crucial role in this process. Efficient breathing activates the body's deep support system, allows the diaphragm to function properly, manages pressure effectively, and enables the core to respond to loads without creating unnecessary tension.

This is why the old advice to "tighten your core" can cause problems. Bracing too much makes it harder to breathe, tires you out, and leaves your muscles feeling tight. If you already have pain, this can make things worse. The diaphragm, pelvic floor, and deep abdominal muscles all work together as a pressure system. When this system works as it should, your body stabilizes itself without extra effort. Breathing and movement begin to work together rather than against each other. Holding your breath during effort can also lead to strain. It raises internal pressure but takes away your body's ability to adapt. It can feel strong in the moment, but it often shows up later as fatigue, tightness, or flare-ups.

Over time, this teaches your nervous system that movement requires tension. When you let your breath guide your stability, strength feels safer. Your movements become smoother, and effort is distributed instead of concentrated in one area.

The Deep Support System

Stability is commonly associated with the abdominal muscles; however, support and movement depend on coordinated activity across many muscle groups. For instance, the deep neck flexors contribute to control and coordination of the head and neck. Research shows that people with neck pain can have altered function of these muscles, and targeted training can improve neuromuscular coordination.

Additionally, the muscles around the shoulder blades also contribute to shoulder and upper-body movement, and scapular stabilization exercises may help improve pain and function in people with chronic neck pain. The gluteal muscles play an important role in controlling the hip and pelvis, and research has found differences in gluteal function in some people with low back pain. Finally, deeper spinal muscles such as the multifidus contribute to control and stability of the spine during movement.[4]

When these muscles go quiet, bigger muscles step in to protect you, and that protection often shows up as stiffness or guarding. The smaller muscles in our body play a crucial role as they provide subtle support, enhance control, and aid the nervous system in relaxing. Unfortunately, pain-focused training often neglects these important muscles in favor of larger, more visible ones. By re-engaging these smaller muscles, we can significantly change how our body manages physical load.

For example, an individual experiencing ongoing neck pain might have well-developed upper trapezius muscles but weak deep neck support. If they only focus on strengthening the already dominant muscles, it could lead to increased tension. Therefore, concentrating on activating the deeper neck muscles often helps alleviate pain, even if overall strength does not improve. This pattern can also be observed in the lower body.

People with strong legs but poor hip control may feel unsteady. By prioritizing coordination instead of solely increasing strength, they can enhance how their movements feel.

Strength Training for Sensitive and Stressed Bodies

Individuals sensitive to pain or stress often benefit from a training approach that emphasizes low loads and high control, as heavy weights and fast tempos can trigger flare-ups, especially in the early stages. By beginning with slow, controlled movements, the nervous system has time to adjust, which helps reduce startle responses and build confidence. Maintaining a steady tempo, therefore, keeps the body organized, while avoiding rushed movements that can lead to protective tension.

Moreover, focusing on varied movement patterns promotes strength relevant to daily life and effectively reduces pain. Lastly, using simple props such as chairs, walls, resistance bands, or towels provides support and feedback without adding undue pressure, further enhancing the training experience.

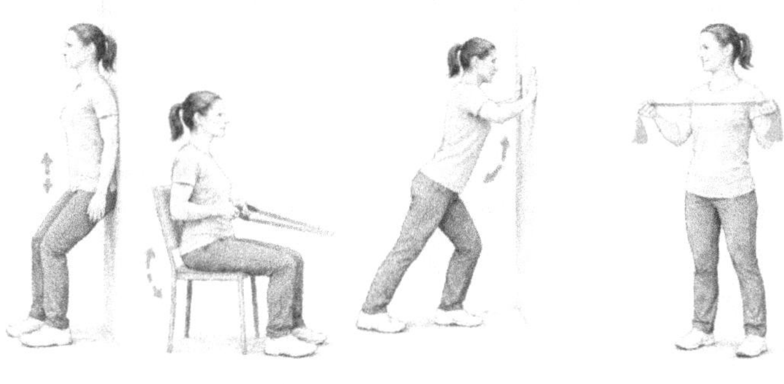

Figure 5.1: Supported strength patterns using props

Strength training helps with pain when you build it with awareness. If you don't challenge yourself enough, your body won't be ready. If you do too much too quickly, your body may tense up, and you might become more fearful. The aim is to add load in a way that feels manageable, repeatable, and predictable.

Pain-safe progress doesn't mean avoiding all discomfort; rather, it's about learning to distinguish between excessive strain and normal effort. Typically, productive discomfort feels dull or like hard work, and it fades quickly after you stop moving. In contrast, harmful pain often feels sharp, sudden, or alarming. It may cause you to hold your breath or urge you to stop immediately, and it can persist or worsen over time. Developing the ability to differentiate between these sensations builds confidence, reduces your perception of threat, and can lessen the sensitivity to pain.

The four basic movement patterns—push, pull, hinge, and squat—are fundamental to many daily activities. Practicing these movements gently and regularly prepares your body for everyday life, not just for workouts.

To create a full-body workout, pick one exercise from each movement type.

Push Movement Patterns

Push movements are important for everyday tasks like standing up, placing objects on high shelves, and reaching out. When the body is sensitive or recovering from pain, these patterns should be reintroduced with support and low load. A good way to start is with a wall push-up. Stand an arm's length from the wall, put your hands on it, and slowly bend and straighten your elbows. Keep your posture upright and breathe smoothly, and if you find yourself holding your breath, the exercise might be too hard. Once this feels comfortable, you can gradually make it harder by adjusting the angle or moving closer to the floor. These variations help you build strength safely before progressing to more traditional exercises, such as bench presses or overhead presses.

In traditional strength training, push movements include horizontal presses, such as push-ups or bench presses, and vertical presses, such as overhead shoulder presses. These exercises primarily target the chest, triceps, and shoulders. When done at the right time and with the right weight, they help build strength that supports everyday activities and long-term health.

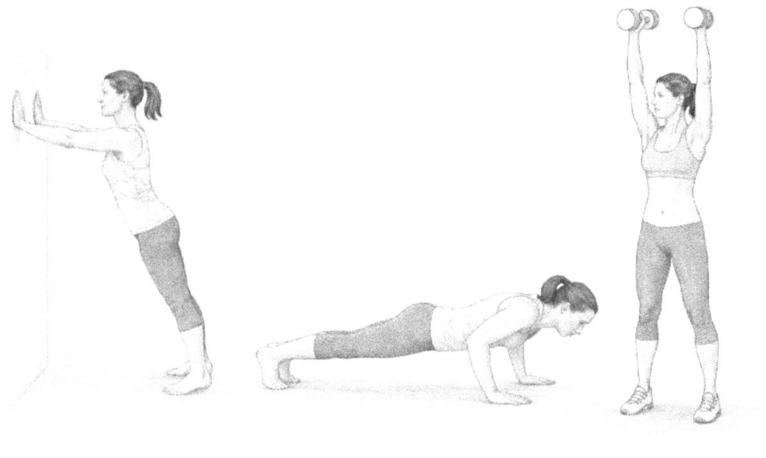

Figure 5.2: Push movement patterns

Pull Movement Patterns

Pulling movements are integral to many daily activities, such as opening drawers, drawing objects closer, or stabilizing the arms while carrying items. However, individuals experiencing pain may avoid these actions due to instability in their shoulders or neck. To safely and progressively improve these movements, one can practice pull patterns with simple tools, such as a resistance band or a towel secured to a door handle. This approach can help regain strength and stability without risking further discomfort.

Start seated or standing with support. When pulling, let the shoulder blades move naturally instead of holding them in a fixed position. Do not forcefully pinch the shoulder blades together. The movement should remain smooth, controlled, and coordinated. If you experience neck tension, the load or speed is likely too high. Practicing pull patterns can improve posture by restoring balanced effort around the shoulders.

In traditional strength training, pull patterns include horizontal pulls, such as rows and seated rows, and vertical pulls, such as pull-ups or lat pull-downs. These exercises primarily target the upper back muscles, including the latissimus dorsi, trapezius, posterior deltoids, and biceps. When performed with appropriate timing and load, pull patterns build strength that supports daily activities and promotes long-term resilience in the shoulders and neck.

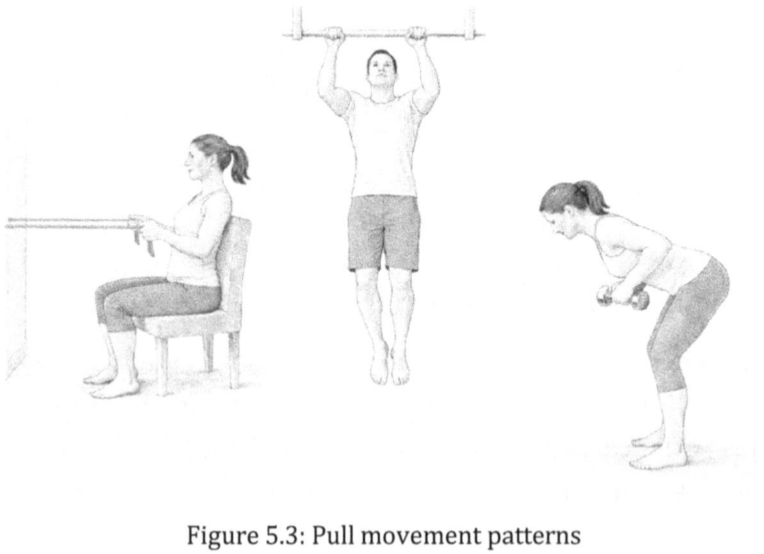

Figure 5.3: Pull movement patterns

Hinge Movement Patterns

Hinge movements prepare the body for bending, lifting, and lowering objects. These patterns shift movement through the hips rather than the spine alone, but they do not eliminate spinal motion entirely. This balanced distribution of motion helps reduce fear and builds confidence in everyday bending tasks. A supported hinge is an effective starting point. Place your hands on your thighs or a chair and slowly fold forward from the hips, letting your spine move naturally within a range that feels good. Use your legs and hips to get back up. The focus is on moving smoothly and keeping control. Many people are surprised to learn that letting the spine move gently makes them less afraid.

You can add light objects as your tolerance grows. The load should feel easy enough that breathing remains calm. As confidence improves, the hinge can be practiced on one leg. This challenges balance and load-sharing without adding weight. Start with a very small range and keep the movement slow. Single-leg work helps the hips and nervous system coordinate more precisely, which often builds trust faster than heavier loads.

In more traditional strength-training contexts, hinge patterns include movements such as deadlifts, hip thrusts, and back extensions. These exercises primarily engage the gluteal, hamstring, and lower back muscles. When introduced progressively and with appropriate load, hinge patterns build strength that transfers directly to daily lifting tasks and long-term resilience of the hips and spine.

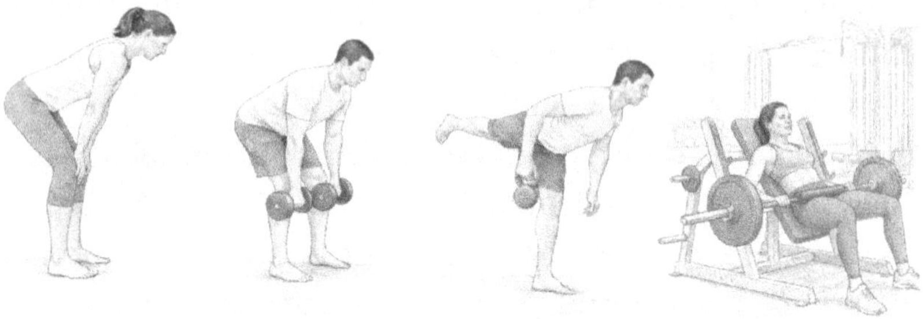

Figure 5.4: Hinge movement patterns

Squat Movement Patterns

Squatting helps with everyday activities like sitting and standing. For pain-sensitive bodies, a chair is an ideal starting point. This pattern allows the legs to take on load in a familiar, controlled way, helping rebuild confidence in movements performed many times each day. Start with a sit-to-stand pattern. Begin by sitting down slowly, then push through your legs to stand, keeping control and breathing steadily. You can use your hands for support first, then reduce this support over time.

At the beginning, focus on moving with control rather than on how deep you squat. A shallow squat is preferable to a deep squat performed with tension. By practicing control, your body can adjust to the movement without causing unnecessary discomfort.

Wall squats are an excellent starting point, particularly for those with knee pain or limited experience. The wall provides support and feedback, helping you maintain proper posture and balance. Slower, controlled movements can also help your nervous system feel more secure. As your strength and confidence improve, you can progress to free-standing squats or sit-to-stand exercises. This gradual approach makes the squat pattern more automatic and applicable to daily activities.

Traditional strength training includes bodyweight squats, weighted squats, single-leg squats, and lunges. These exercises engage the gluteal muscles, quadriceps, and hamstrings. When the load is held in front of the body, or when the heels are elevated, the movement tends to emphasize the quadriceps. Conversely, when the weight is positioned on the back, the exercise typically becomes more glute-dominant.

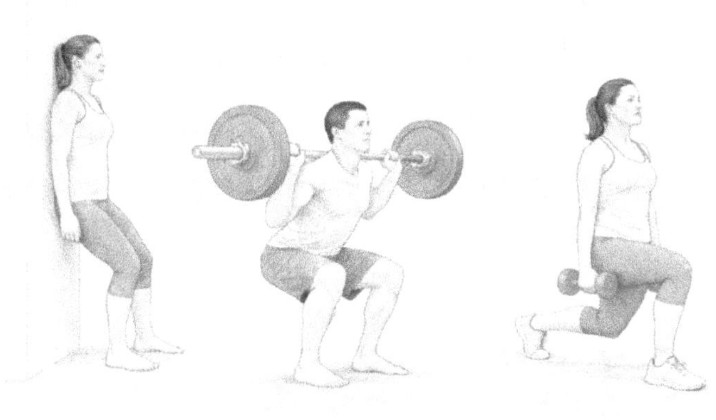

Figure 5.5: Squat movement patterns

When to Stop an Exercise

Stop exercising if you experience a sharp increase in pain, have difficulty breathing, or notice a rapid decline in your movement. Feeling tired is normal, but feeling alarmed is not. If any discomfort subsides within a few minutes and you feel fine later that day and the next morning, then the intensity of your exercise was likely appropriate for you. Reducing the intensity is not a failure; it's a smart approach to continue making progress.

The 15-Minute Strength and Stability Builder

This routine combines strength, stability, and movement coordination using all the main patterns: pull, push, squat, and hinge. You can do it three to five times a week, or even daily if you keep the intensity low. The focus is on improving coordination, breathing, and control, not on pushing yourself as hard as possible. Move slowly, pay attention to your breath and how your body feels. Take breaks when you need to and stop before you get too tired to keep good form.

The repetition ranges provided below are guidelines only. You can perform fewer repetitions if discomfort or pain appears, or more if the movement feels easy and you want to gently increase muscular engagement. The main thing is to pay attention to your body and not worry too much about the numbers.

Scapular Retraction: A Pull for Postural Strength

The purpose of this movement is to restore coordinated shoulder blade motion, improve stability, and prepare the shoulders for pushing, pulling, and overhead activities. It primarily engages the following muscles:

- Middle and lower trapezius
- Rhomboids
- Posterior deltoid
- Rotator cuff, especially the infraspinatus and teres minor

Together, these muscles help guide the shoulder blades into a stable position, allowing the upper back to support healthy posture and efficient arm movement.

Level 1: Bodyweight Scapular Retraction

Stand upright with elbows bent at 90 degrees and palms facing up. Keep your lower back neutral. Gently draw your shoulder blades together and slightly downward to open the chest. Move your thumbs away from your body and toward your back. Keep your neck relaxed. Return slowly to the starting position.

Perform 8 to 12 slow repetitions for 2 to 3 sets, and keep focusing on slow, controlled movements, and ensure you actively squeeze your shoulder blades together.

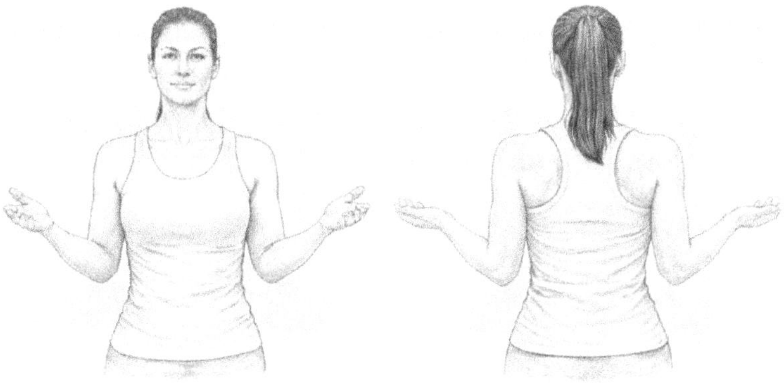

Figure 5.6: Scapular retraction

Level 2: Band Pull-Apart or Band Row

To perform the exercise, start by holding a light elastic band at chest height. Pull the band apart or carry out a controlled row, making sure to initiate the movement with your shoulder blades before engaging your arms. Aim for 8 to 12 slow repetitions, completing 2 to 3 sets.

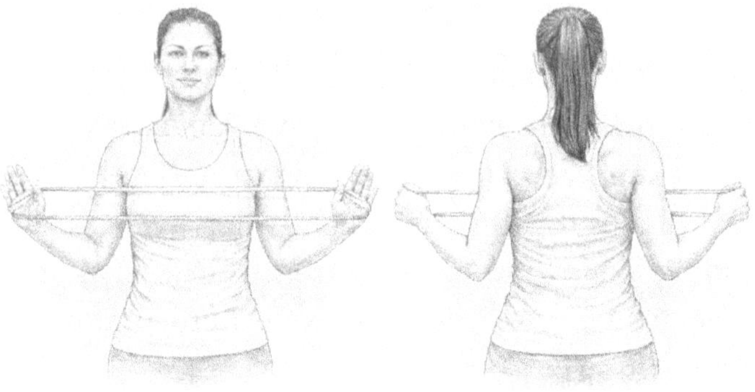

Figure 5.7: Band pull-apart shoulder retraction

Level 3: Dumbbell Row (Supported)

For this exercise, place one hand on a bench or chair for support. With the other arm, row a light dumbbell, allowing your shoulder blade to move naturally instead of holding it in place. Aim for 2 to 3 sets, performing 8 to 12 slow repetitions each time.

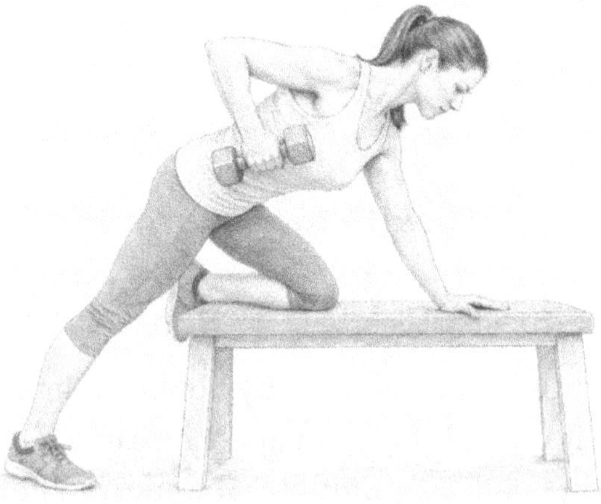

Figure 5.8: Dumbbell row

These activities help in reducing neck and shoulder strain and improve efficiency in all upper-body movements.

Level 4: Assisted or Full Pull-Up

To build full-body pulling strength and enhance advanced scapular control, it's essential to engage the arms, trunk, and hips. Therefore, this level of training is designed to improve shoulder stability under heavier loads. It also develops the strength necessary for activities like climbing, hanging, and lifting by engaging the following muscles:

- Latissimus dorsi
- Lower and middle trapezius
- Rhomboids
- Biceps brachii
- Brachialis and brachioradialis

To perform this exercise, hang from a bar with your hands slightly wider than shoulder-width apart. Gently draw your shoulder blades down and back, then pull your body upward until your chin approaches or clears the bar. Lower yourself slowly and with control, allowing your shoulder blades to move naturally at the bottom. Maintain smooth, steady breathing throughout the movement. Avoid excessive neck tension and prevent swinging.

Progressions:

- **Band-assisted pull-up:** Loop a resistance band around the bar and place your foot or knee in the band to decrease resistance.
- **Jumping pull-up with slow eccentric:** Jump to the top position, then lower yourself slowly over 3 to 5 seconds.
- **Full pull-up:** Use only your bodyweight, maintaining control throughout the entire movement.

Dosage:

For optimal results, aim for 3 to 8 repetitions in 2 to 3 sets, adjusting based on your fitness level. Focus on maintaining proper form rather than simply trying to complete more repetitions. Additionally, ensure you take adequate rest between sets to recover effectively.

Key focus points:

To initiate the movement effectively, focus on engaging your shoulder blades rather than relying solely on your arms. It's essential to maintain control during the lowering phase, as this aspect is just as crucial as the pulling motion itself.

Remember, this stage represents the pinnacle of the pull progression and should be introduced only after the previous levels have been mastered, ensuring they are stable, controlled, and pain-free.

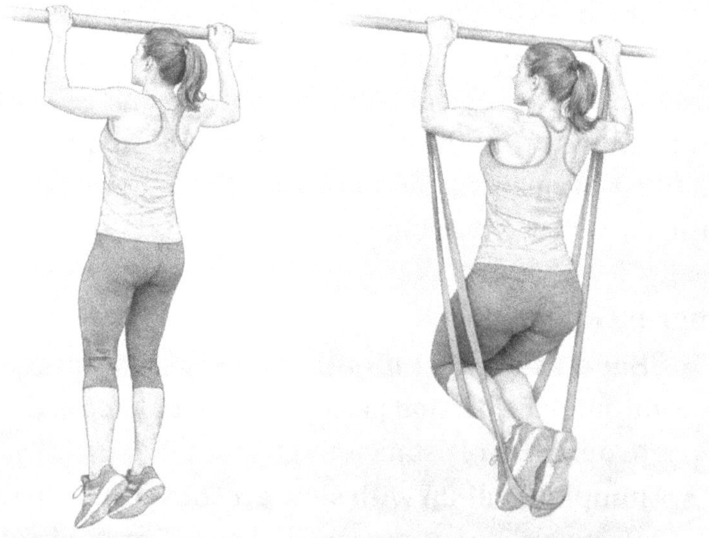

Figure 5.9: Assisted and full pull-up

Supported Squat or Sit-Stand: Squat Movement Pattern for Lower-Body Strength

To build a strong foundation for your lower body, it's essential to focus on movements that mimic everyday activities. Enhancing your leg strength and coordination can significantly improve tasks like sitting, standing, and navigating stairs.

The primary muscles engaged in this process include:

- Quadriceps
- Gluteus maximus
- Hamstrings
- Deep trunk stabilizers

Before progressing through the levels, focus on moving with control and working within a pain-free range. Each stage builds on the previous one, so it's important to feel stable and confident before advancing.

Level 1: Sit-to-Stand

To perform this exercise safely and effectively, begin by sitting down in a chair, then stand up slowly and in a controlled manner. You can use your hands on your thighs or the armrests for added support. Aim for 6 to 10 slow repetitions, completing 2 to 3 sets. Remember to prioritize control over depth throughout the movement.

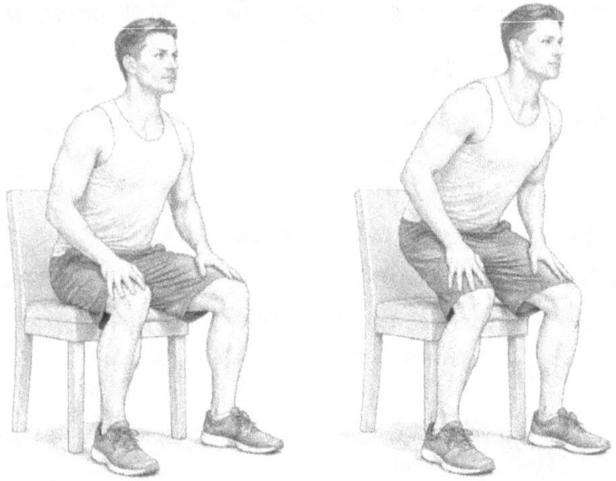

Figure 5.10: Sit-to-stand

Level 2: Free Squat (Partial Range of Movement) or Wall Sit

To perform effective lower-body exercises, start by removing any chair and transitioning into a squat. Aim to squat to a comfortable depth while maintaining your balance and steady breathing. For those experiencing knee pain, wall sits are an excellent alternative. To do a wall sit, begin by standing with your back against a wall, then step forward about four feet so that when you lower into the position, your hips and knees form a 90-degree angle. For an easier variation, you can stop just before reaching this depth.

Initially, hold the position for 15 to 30 seconds, gradually working your way up to one minute or longer as your strength improves. Remember to maintain steady breathing throughout the exercise and keep your upper body relaxed for the best results.

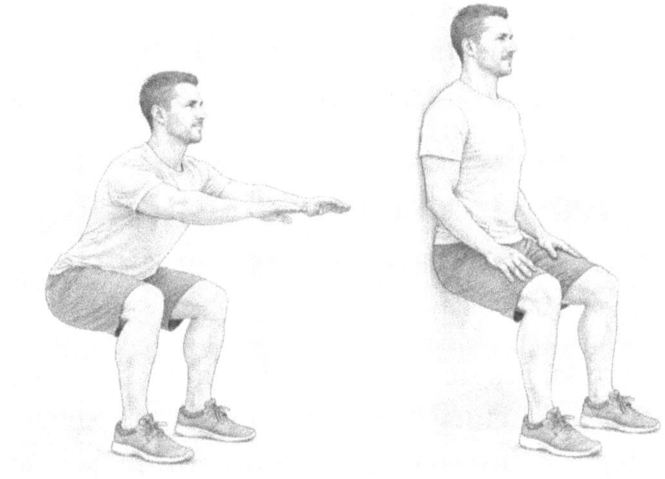

Figure 5.11: Free squat and wall sit

Level 3: Loaded squat

For a loaded squat, hold a light dumbbell or kettlebell in front of your chest, or use two light dumbbells at your sides. Then, aim to perform 6 to 10 repetitions for 2 to 3 sets, focusing on maintaining control over the depth of your squat.

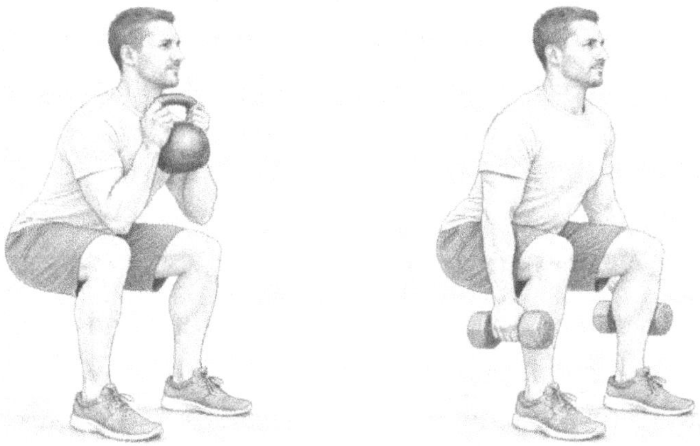

Figure 5.12: Loaded squat

Squatting is beneficial for restoring confidence in knee and hip movements, ultimately leading to improved functionality in daily activities.

Wall Push-Up to Floor Push-Up: Push Movement Pattern for Upper-Body Strength

This exercise progression is designed to help you build upper-body strength while maintaining proper shoulder and trunk stability throughout the movement. By starting with the wall push-up and transitioning to the floor push-up, you can gradually increase the intensity and challenge your muscles more directly.

It involves the following muscles:

- Pectoralis major
- Triceps
- Anterior deltoid
- Serratus anterior (important for scapular control)

Before beginning the levels, focus on maintaining a straight body line, engaging your core, and allowing your shoulder blades to move naturally. Progress gradually, ensuring each level feels controlled and pain-free before moving on.

Level 1: Wall push-up

Place your hands on the wall and keep your body straight or slightly inclined. If you stand farther from the wall, rise onto your toes. Lower your body slowly, then press back as you exhale gently.

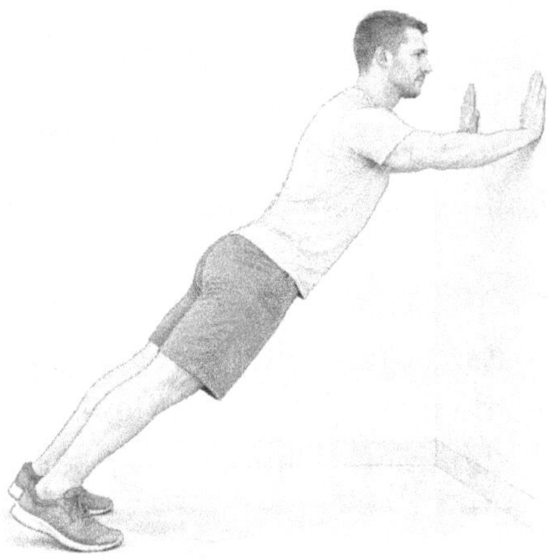

Figure 5.13: Wall push-up (slightly harder variation with the incline)

Level 2: Incline Push-Up

To perform the exercise with increased resistance, place your hands on a bench, chair, or counter. Aim to complete 8 to 12 repetitions for a total of 2 to 3 sets.

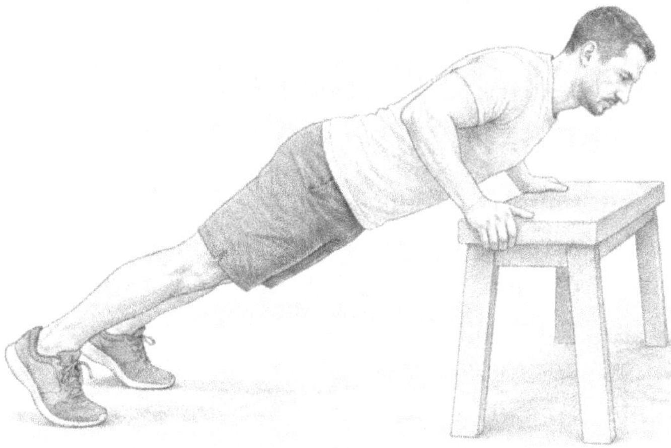

Figure 5.14: Incline push-up

Level 3: Floor Push-Up

As your strength improves, progress to knee or full push-ups. Aim to perform 6 to 10 repetitions for 2 to 3 sets. Remember to allow your shoulder blades to move naturally throughout the exercise.

Pressing strength is essential as it enables effective pushing movements, assists with rising from the floor, and helps protect the shoulders by strengthening the muscles of the scapula and shoulder (rotator cuff, serratus anterior, rhomboids, trapezius).

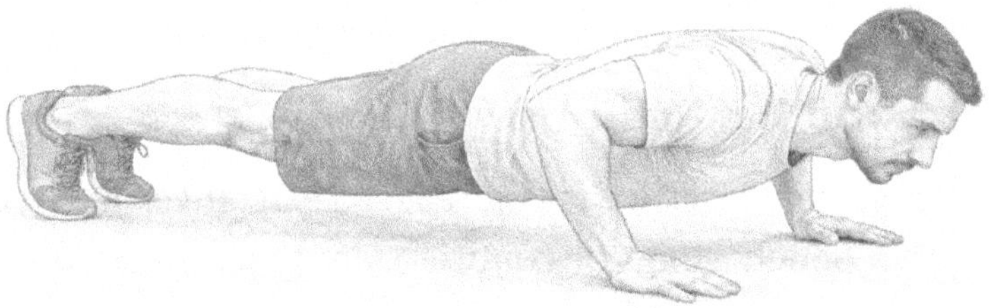

Figure 5.15: Floor push-up

Hip Hinge: Hinge Pattern for Posterior Chain Strength

Build strength and confidence for safe bending, lifting, and carrying by mastering the hip hinge movement. This pattern emphasizes proper loading through the hips while maintaining a stable spine, helping to protect the lower back. Primary muscles involved:

- Gluteus maximus
- Hamstrings
- Erector spinae
- Deep spinal stabilizers

Level 1: Supported Hip Hinge

Place your hands on your thighs or hold a light object close to your body. Hinge at the hips, maintaining a comfortable and natural spinal position.

Level 2: Loaded Hinge

Hold a light dumbbell or kettlebell close to your body. Aim to perform 8 to 12 controlled repetitions for 2 to 3 sets.

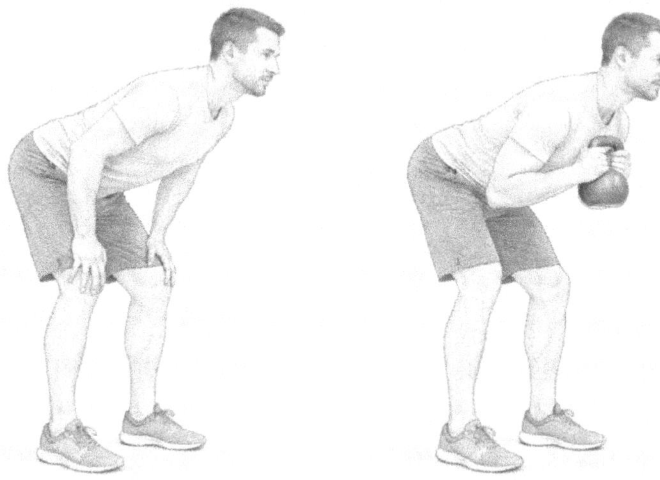

Figure 5.16: Supported hip hinge and loaded hinge

Level 3: Single-Leg Hinge

Lift one foot off the ground to enhance balance and increase the load on a single leg. Hold a dumbbell in the opposite hand of the grounded leg. Ensure that the movement is driven by the hip rather than the back, keeping your back straight throughout. Distribute your weight evenly on the grounded foot, taking care to prevent the knee from collapsing inward.

Aim for 6 to 10 controlled repetitions across 2 to 3 sets, emphasizing smooth and deliberate movements.

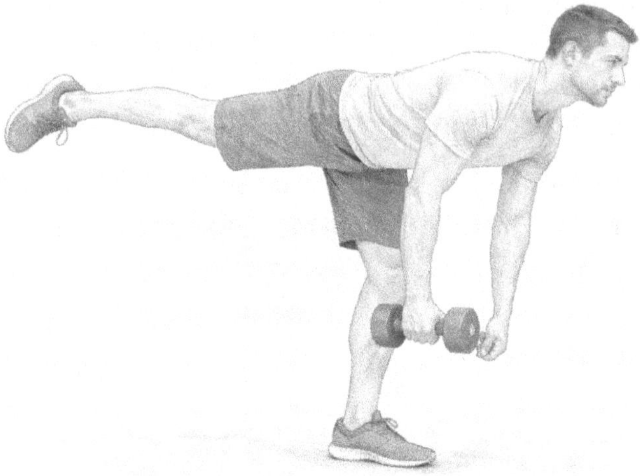

Figure 5.17: Single-leg hinge

In short, learning to control how your spine moves can make you more resilient. Practicing the single-leg hip hinge helps you build stability, strength, and confidence for everyday tasks.

Now, let's move onto glute section.

Glute Bridge with Breath Coordination

Enhance coordination among the hips, pelvis, and breathing while strengthening the posterior chain. This exercise helps reinforce efficient movement patterns and spinal stability.

Primary muscles involved:

- Gluteus maximus
- Hamstrings
- Deep abdominal muscles

Before progressing through the levels, focus on smooth, controlled breathing and maintaining a stable pelvis. Each phase should feel steady and well-coordinated rather than forced.

Level 1: Basic Glute Bridge

Lie on your back with your knees bent. Inhale, then exhale as you lift your hips. Inhale again as you lower your hips. For greater hamstring engagement, move your feet farther away and lift your toes. This position should resemble a reverse plank.

Perform 8 to 12 controlled repetitions for 2 to 3 sets.

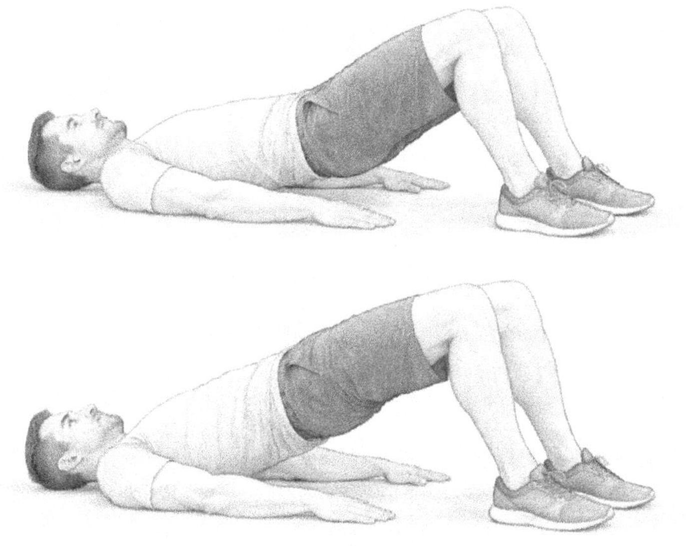

Figure 5.18: Basic glute bridge

Level 2: Pause Bridge

Hold at the top for 30 to 60 seconds, breathing steadily, keeping the glutes engaged but without tensing the back or shoulders.

Level 3: Single-leg Bridge

To perform this exercise, start by lifting one foot slightly off the floor while keeping your pelvis stable. It's important to avoid allowing your pelvis to drop as you raise your leg. Aim for 6 to 10 repetitions, and complete 2 to 3 sets.

Remember to keep the movement steady and controlled for the best results.

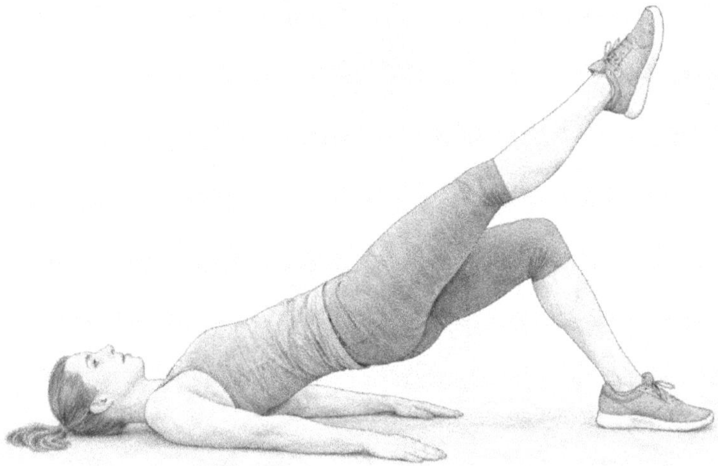

Figure 5.19: Single-leg bridge

This pattern helps you coordinate your breath, pelvis, and trunk, improving both stability and the efficiency of your movement.

How to Use This Routine

This routine enhances overall strength by emphasizing coordinated movements instead of isolating specific muscles. If you notice feelings of calmness, warmth, and increased confidence after your session, it indicates that the routine is effective. You don't need to exert maximum effort to achieve strength; as you become accustomed to the exercises, you can gradually increase the number of repetitions, incorporate resistance, or explore more challenging variations.

Example

After a few weeks of this kind of training, many people find that pain no longer controls their choices. They might still notice some sensations, but these feel less important. Movements that used to seem risky now feel doable. Recovery gets better. Building strength does not remove pain directly, but it changes how the body handles stress.

Always prioritize control before attempting greater challenges. Remember, strength developed safely is more sustainable. Gradually, you will be able to increase intensity and range of motion to challenge yourself, transforming structured movements into natural and fluid motion.

Strength In the Real World

Strength works best when it fits naturally into your daily life. Many people think a good exercise plan should always give steady results, but chronic pain doesn't always follow this pattern. Your ability to exercise depends on how well you sleep, your stress, your mood, and how well you recover, not just on your training. All of these factors affect how your nervous system responds to physical effort.[5]

Because of this, strength training might help one week but make symptoms worse the next, even if you do the same exercises. When you are more stressed or not sleeping well, your body focuses on keeping balance. Thus, adding more exercise at these times can prompt your body to protect itself rather than adapt. This shows why timing matters in strength training, not that strength training itself is harmful.

I have experienced this firsthand while climbing. On some days, training felt strong, coordinated, and confident. On others, despite equal effort, nothing seemed to work. My grip tightened too early, my breathing became shallow, and I could not relax. Forcing strength only increased my tension. What helped was stepping back and allowing myself to reset. When I calmed down, my strength returned naturally.

The earlier steps in this book address this process. Calming yourself, increasing awareness, releasing tension, and improving movement all contribute to building strength. Once you master these fundamentals, gaining strength becomes more natural. Movements become easier, breathing improves under pressure, and your body responds as expected.

Even with good timing and steady progress, flare-ups can still happen. This is normal. A flare does not mean something is wrong. It is just information.

A flare-up often reflects a temporary mismatch between capacity and demand rather than structural damage.[6] High stress, poor sleep, illness, or sudden changes in your routine can all lower your tolerance. When this happens, it is usually better not to stop moving completely. Instead, you can adjust by lowering the intensity, moving less, slowing down, or doing fewer repetitions. This keeps your body active without making it feel threatened. Learning to handle flare-ups builds confidence. Over time, people stop seeing pain spikes as a sign of weakness. They start to see them as useful signals. This change often reduces fear and tension, which can help lower overall pain.

As you continue strength training, you'll likely notice some small but important changes. Everyday tasks start to feel easier, and movements like standing, lifting, carrying, and walking come more naturally. You don't have to think about your body as much. You might still notice some sensations, but they don't feel as urgent. You recover more quickly, and your body settles down faster after stress. This is when you really see the value of strength. It doesn't remove all discomfort, but it changes how you experience it. With a stronger body, the same challenges seem less threatening. Daily life feels more manageable and less overwhelming.

Over time, this physical change supports a psychological one. Long-standing pain often shapes identity. Many people begin to see themselves as careful, limited, or fragile. Strength challenges this identity through experience rather than reassurance. Each calm, controlled repetition sends a new message: your body can handle a load. It can adapt. It is not as fragile as it once felt. This shift does not happen overnight. It builds quietly through consistency. Eventually, strength stops feeling like a task that must be carefully managed and becomes a background support system. Movement becomes something the body does rather than something that has to be negotiated. This is the real aim of this step. Not maximal strength. Not a perfect technique. But a body that feels capable enough to meet daily demands without constant protection.

Final Thoughts

As we're closing this chapter, it is important to remember that strength isn't about controlling or dominating your body. It's about cooperation. When you feel capable, your nervous system can relax. As you relax, pain often feels less urgent. This step prepares you for the last phase: applying what you've learned in your daily life, under stress, and in movement beyond exercise. In the next chapter, we'll focus on integration and how to live in a way that truly supports the changes you've made.

CHAPTER 6

Regulate and Restore

Your spine can't relax until your mind feels safe.

At this point, your relationship with pain has changed. You might still have symptoms, but they no longer dictate your choices. Moving feels more predictable, and flare-ups make more sense. Your body seems less fragile. Even as you progress, tension can return under stress, pain may flare with strong emotions, or the body might tighten for no clear reason. This doesn't mean the earlier steps failed. Rather, it points to the final piece of the puzzle: helping your nervous system truly feel safe.

If the nervous system hasn't learned to relax during stress, physical progress will always seem unfinished. You might have stronger muscles, better movement, and easier posture. But if your mind stays alert, your body remains tense. Therefore, regulation isn't just about calming yourself instantly; it's about making calm possible.

When the nervous system no longer feels threatened, your body can finally rest, heal, and adjust. This process is closely tied to movement and strength, as they mutually support one another. Without proper regulation, your body expends unnecessary energy and struggles to maintain balance. However, once regulation is established, everything you've worked on becomes more manageable and easier to sustain.

How Anxiety Makes Pain Signals Stronger

Pain does not always reflect the actual condition of your tissues. Instead, it is a protective response shaped by your surroundings and feelings. Anxiety can strongly affect this process.[1] When you feel anxious, your brain becomes more alert and focuses on possible dangers. You pay closer attention to sensations, and things that would normally seem harmless may start to feel threatening.

This state is sometimes called the brain's protective mode. Here, your nervous system prioritizes survival over comfort. Your muscles stay a bit tense, your breathing gets shallower, and your heart rate becomes less steady. You may notice pain more easily and start watching your body for any signs of problems. A small ache in your back might feel like a warning, and a usual tightness in your neck could seem like a sign that pain is coming. Your mind may jump to conclusions before your body has a chance to react normally.

As you can see, fear amplifies this process, playing a significant role in the way our bodies respond. When pain lasts for a long time, the brain begins to expect harm from certain sensations and reacts quickly.[2] This early reaction can actually cause symptoms people are worried about. This does not mean the pain is made up. Instead, it shows the system is working too hard to protect you. Just telling yourself that you are safe often isn't enough. If your body remains tense and your breathing is tight, your nervous system will continue to react negatively. It's essential to cultivate a genuine sense of safety, not just think about it. When you calm your system, it reduces your alertness, making the same feelings appear less frightening. Pain signals may diminish not because your body has undergone a change, but because your system no longer feels the need to sound the alarm.

Modern life keeps our nervous system on high alert. News about disasters, scrolling through social media, worries about money, or being constantly connected can all trigger stress, even when there's nothing immediate to act on. Although our brains can distinguish between physical and emotional threats, both can activate similar stress-response systems in the body. Researchers refer to this as "toxic stress," which is activation without effective action, because both trigger the same survival responses.[3] "Neuroception" is the ongoing process in which your nervous system scans your environment, relationships, and internal state to determine if you are safe. [4] The body can become hypersensitive as a result of trauma or prolonged stress, leading it to perceive danger even in safe situations or to remain reactive long after threats have passed.

This reaction is not a character flaw but rather an adaptive response that can become unhelpful over time. Many people notice that their pain often intensifies in anticipation of stressful events such as giving a presentation, having a difficult conversation, or facing a looming deadline—rather than during the event itself. Symptoms may emerge hours or even days in advance, highlighting how the body reacts to the anticipation of stress rather than an actual injury. After the event concludes, these symptoms typically fade on their own. This perspective aligns with understanding pain as a prediction, not merely a sign of physical harm.

Rebuilding Safety through Your Body

Most traditional methods try to change your thoughts. Somatic work, on the other hand, helps your nervous system remember what safety feels like in your body. Your nervous system learns through experience, not just by being told. To truly learn, your body needs new, safe experiences.

Simple Ways to Feel Safer

- **Grounding and Orientation:** Take a slow look around you, noticing the colors, shapes, and textures in your environment. Feel how your feet connect to the ground and how your body is supported. Say out loud five things you can see, four things you can hear, and three things you can feel.
- **Breath as a Safety Signal:** Place one hand on your chest and the other on your belly. Let your breath move gently in and out of your belly. Try the "safety sigh": take a normal inhale, a small second inhale, and a slow exhale with an "ahh" sound.
- **Building Body Awareness:** Practice gentle body scans and simply notice sensations without trying to change anything. Pay attention to areas of tension and take a moment to acknowledge them. Shift your focus between tense spots and calmer areas to enhance awareness and regulation.
- **Creating Micro-Moments of Safety:** Use small, comforting actions to signal safety to your nervous system. Wrap yourself in a soft blanket, hold a warm cup and feel its heat, or listen to calming music. Step outside for fresh air or take a short walk, and engage in gentle stretches or yoga poses.

- **Nervous System Regulation:** Activities like humming or gentle singing can stimulate vagal tone. Short periods of cold exposure or contrast therapy can improve vagal tone, boost resilience, and reduce inflammation.[5] Gentle self-massage around the ears and jaw, along with slow, mindful movement, can further support nervous system regulation.
- **Inner Child and Safety Visualization:** The brain responds to vivid imagery in ways similar to real experiences.[6] Guided visualization can help establish a sense of safety within your nervous system. Consider visualizing a place where you feel safe, supported, and held. Speak gently to your inner child, reassuring them: "You're safe now. I'm here with you."

These practices remind you that safety is not just an external condition but something you can cultivate within yourself. Even brief, consistent efforts can strengthen resilience, calm the nervous system, and foster a deeper sense of well-being.

Emotional Muscle Tension

Emotions are not just in the mind. They also show up in the body. Each emotional state alters muscle tone, posture, and breathing. These reactions happen automatically. With time, they can become habits, even if the original emotion is gone.[7] Anger often appears in the jaw, neck, and shoulders. People may clench their teeth, pull their head back a little, and stiffen their upper body. This tension can persist long after the anger fades, especially if it is held in or left unaddressed.

Worry often shows up in the chest and ribs. Breathing gets shallow and tight, and the rib cage moves less. The body stays a bit tense, almost bracing for something. Over time, this can limit movement and put more strain on the spine and neck. The chest may feel heavier, the head may drift forward, and movement can become smaller and slower. While this posture can feel protective in the short term, prolonged collapse increases the load on certain tissues and reinforces fatigue.[8]

These patterns are not errors but adaptations. They reflect your nervous system's state. When these responses persist, pain may develop as muscles remain tense, breathing becomes shallow, and movement is limited. Even in calm situations, your nervous system may still perceive threat. Forcing your posture or overstretching can lead to increased resistance. Your body will only relax when it feels secure. Remember that recovery is a gradual process. Prioritize awareness, gentle movements, and relaxed breathing; there's no need to push yourself.

Emotional Tension Mapping Exercise (3 to 5 Minutes)

Find a comfortable position, whether sitting or standing, and consider closing your eyes if it feels right. Turn your attention to your jaw, neck, chest, ribs, and shoulders. Take a brief pause and ask yourself, "What am I truly feeling at this moment?" There's no need to overanalyze or label the emotion, just acknowledging it can help alleviate its intensity.

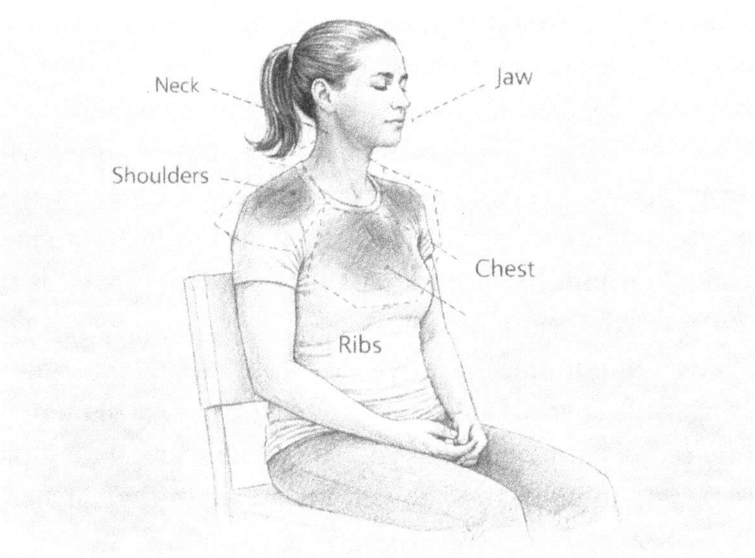

Figure 6.1: Emotional tension mapping exercise

Meditation for People Who Hate Meditation

Many people who live with pain find meditation frustrating or unrealistic. Sitting still can make symptoms feel worse. Closing your eyes might make you more anxious, and trying to "clear your mind" often backfires. Thoughts get busier, and your body stays tense. The real issue is not meditation itself, but how it is often taught. You do not need to sit still for long periods, remain silent, or use special postures. What matters are brief, repeatable moments when you shift your attention from pain to the present. These moments help break the stress cycle and allow your nervous system to reset. For those sensitive to pain, shorter practices are often more effective.[9] Even 60 seconds of focused attention, repeated a few times a day, can help your nervous system return to a normal state. Over time, this can reduce background tension and make you less reactive.

Focused attention is the most basic type of meditation. You pick a neutral anchor and keep your attention on it for a short time. This anchor might be something you feel, hear, or see. The aim is not to block out thoughts, but to notice when your mind wanders and gently bring it back. This process is important because each time you return your focus, you help retrain your mind. Every return tells your body that it is safe to be in the present moment.

Micro-mindfulness uses this idea in daily life. Instead of setting aside special time to meditate, you use small moments that already happen during your day, like waiting for a page to load, standing in the shower, or sitting in the car before driving. These moments are easy to miss, but they can be great chances to practice meditation. If you do this often, these short breaks can help lower stress on your nervous system. Your body will spend less time feeling tense and more time in a state that allows it to recover.

60-Second Attention Reset

Find a comfortable position, sitting or standing. Pick one thing to focus on, like your feet touching the floor, your breath moving in your ribs, or a steady sound nearby. Keep your attention on that for one minute. If your mind wanders, simply notice it and bring your focus back. Let everything else stay as it is. After a minute, go on with your day.

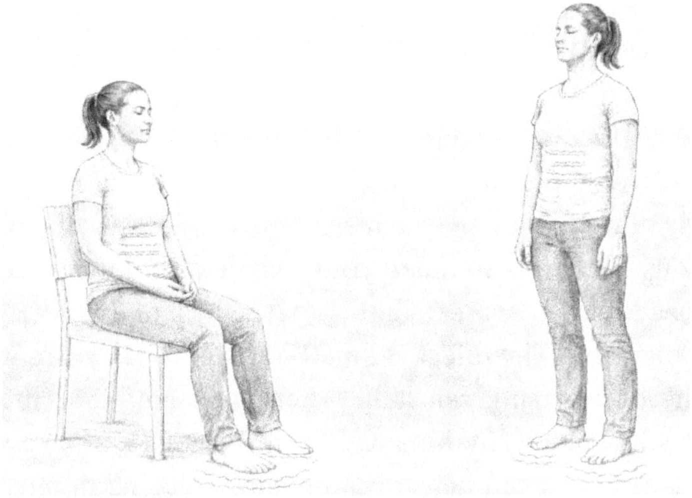

Figure 6.2: Simple focused-attention grounding

Why Does This Work for Pain

Paying close attention helps the brain worry less about possible threats.[10] When you focus on the present, your mind is less likely to look for future dangers. Your muscles may relax a bit, and your breathing often becomes deeper naturally. As a result, pain sensitivity can start to decrease. This shift happens without forcing yourself to relax. Many people find that while pain may not go away during these practices, it feels less overwhelming. Noticing this change is often the first sign that the technique is helping.

Breathwork as Emotional Regulation

Breathing is one of the few things the body does that can be automatic and changed. When used gently and consistently, this is a very useful tool for regulation. When you're stressed, your breathing quickens and deepens, which can make your nervous system more alert.[11] This makes small aches feel louder, almost like turning up the volume on your body's alarm system.

With breathing techniques, your breathing can slow down on its own. You don't have to hold your breath or try any extreme methods. Instead, practice breathing more slowly and taking longer pauses. One easy way to calm your nervous system is to make your exhale a bit longer. Longer exhales help activate calming pathways and lower your overall stress. The effect is small but steady. Box breathing, on the other hand, can help when your emotions feel too strong. Its steady rhythm gives your nervous system a sense of order, which can be especially useful during moments of stress or pain. Breathwork should always feel helpful and safe. If you start to feel dizzy, anxious, or uncomfortable, just go back to your normal breathing.

Long-Exhale Breathing Practice

To begin, find a comfortable position by either sitting or lying down. Take a deep breath in through your nose for a count of four, allowing your abdomen to expand fully. Then, exhale gently through your mouth for a count of six to release any tension. Remember not to force your breath; it should feel natural and soothing. Repeat this process for one to three minutes. This breathing practice is especially beneficial in the evening or after experiencing stressful events, helping you unwind and relax.

Box Breathing

Box breathing is a technique that can help ground and calm the mind. Begin by inhaling for a count of four, filling your lungs completely. Once you reach four counts, hold your breath for another four counts to allow your body to stabilize.

Next, exhale slowly for four counts, releasing any tension or stress. After exhaling, hold your breath for 4 counts before starting the cycle over. This method can be repeated for one to three minutes, creating a sense of tranquility and focus as you practice.

Use this when feeling overwhelmed or mentally scattered.

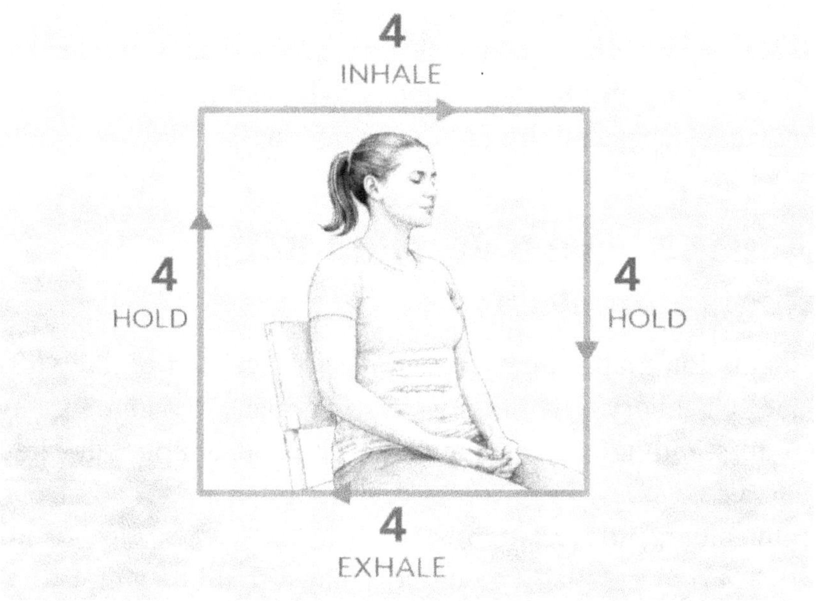

Figure 6.3: Box breathing visual guide

Real-World Example

Many individuals find that their pain intensifies at night as the day winds down. As daytime distractions fade, accumulated stress often becomes more apparent. Engaging in gentle evening breathwork can help ease this pattern by calming the body's overall arousal, allowing the system to settle rather than eliminating the sensation entirely.

The Interaction Between Breath and Movement

Breathwork is most effective when integrated with gentle movement. Slow, controlled breathing during activities such as walking, stretching, or floor exercises promotes a sense of physical safety.[12] Even something as simple as taking a slow walk around your room while paying attention to your breath can help your body feel safe as you move. This approach demonstrates that it is possible to move while maintaining a state of calm. For this reason, previous steps emphasized breathing, as it connects movement, physical strength, and emotional stability.

Action Steps: Daily Mind-Body Regulation Plan

Regulation matters most when it becomes part of daily life, not just theory. The nervous system doesn't change just by understanding it. It changes with practice. Simple, repeated signals of safety help the system respond better to stress, movement, and sensation.[13]

Therefore, a daily regulation plan should be simple, not long or complicated. Keeping things easy helps prevent stress, which is the main goal. Try to include short breaks during the day so your system can relax before stress builds up.

Most people find it helpful to have three simple tools: one for acute stress, one for ongoing tension during the day, and one for relaxing in the evening. Using these tools together helps prevent overload instead of dealing with it later.

Tool 1: Interrupting Acute Stress

Acute stress is a normal part of life. Things like a tough email, sudden pain, a tense conversation, or an urgent request can quickly trigger a stress response. In these moments, the aim is not to get rid of the stress but to stop it from getting worse. Breathing or attention exercises work well for this. They are fast and can be done anywhere. Taking a slow, deep breath with a longer exhale, or briefly focusing on your body, can help interrupt the stress response before it builds. These tools work best when used early. If you use them at the first sign of tension, you can prevent your body from fully entering stress mode.

Tool 2: Reducing Background Tension During the Day

Background tension can sneak up on you. Sitting for long periods, staying focused for hours, dealing with emotions, and not moving much all add up. If you don't take breaks, this tension builds and can make you more sensitive to pain by the end of the day. Gentle movement and paying attention to your body are the best ways to balance out tension.

You don't need to set aside time for full workouts. Simple things like changing your posture, taking short walks, gently moving your neck or lower back, or taking a few deep breaths can help keep your body feeling good. What matters most is how often you do these resets, not how hard you work. Taking just one minute every hour to move or breathe is better than waiting until the end of the day when you're already tired.

Try connecting these quick resets to things you already do, like getting up for water, finishing a task, or sitting down after standing. These moments can remind you to take a short break.

Tool 3: Evening Wind Down and Recovery

Many people notice pain more in the evening. As the day's distractions fade, the nervous system begins to process the stress that has accumulated. If your body has been tense all day, this shift can feel uncomfortable instead of relaxing. A simple wind-down routine signals to your body that it is safe to rest.[14]

You do not need anything complicated. The most helpful steps are to lower stimulation, breathe more slowly, and move gently. Try dimming the lights, using screens less, and slowing down your activities. Gentle floor stretches or calm breathing can help your body recover.

Remember, consistency matters more than duration. Just five minutes each night has been shown to improve sleep quality and reduce physiological arousal.[15]

Boost your energy and calm your mind with this easy daily regulation plan:

Time of Day	Activity	Quick Tip / Fun Twist
Morning	Begin your day calmly	Take 2 minutes to breathe slowly or do a mini body scan. Try gentle neck and lower back stretches to shake off morning stiffness. 🌞
Midday	Take short breaks	Pause 1–2 times during the day. Do a 60-second focus exercise, take slow breaths, or go for a mini walk. Keep your spine happy! 🏃
Evening	Focus on recovery	Slow your breathing, dim the lights, and let your body relax. Gentle movement or just being still works, whatever feels good! 🌙

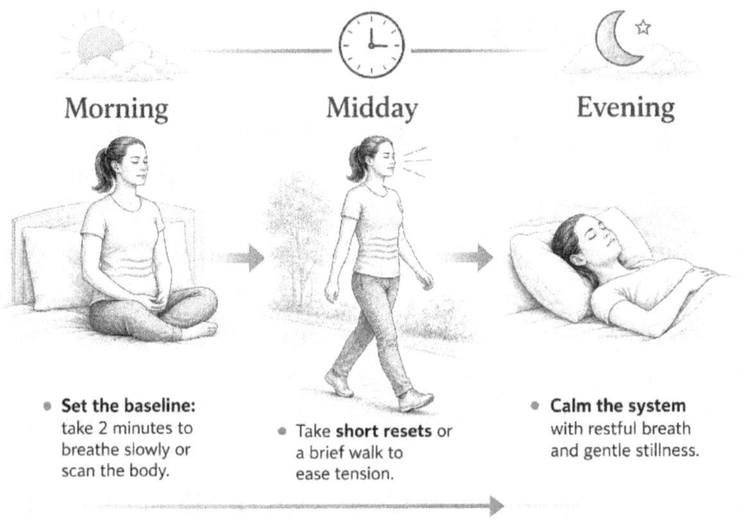

Figure 6.4: Simple daily regulation flow

Mental Reset Moments

Regulation is easier when it is part of everyday life rather than a separate task. These moments are already there. You just need to notice them. Brushing teeth. Waiting while your food cooks. Standing in the shower. Sitting in the car before driving. If you use these moments for short regulation exercises, your nervous system gets regular practice throughout the day. With time, you'll notice it becomes easier to calm down on your own.

Final Thoughts

This final step does not replace movement, release, alignment, or strength; it helps these benefits last longer. Without regulation, the nervous system can revert to protective mode under stress, and old habits may return. With regulation, your body maintains the movement, strength, and confidence you've gained. Many people notice that flare-ups are less intense and shorter. Others may still feel pain, but it feels less threatening. Both are signs of progress.

The goal is not a body that never reacts, but one that can recover. As regulation improves, pain feels less intense. Sensations are interpreted as information, not urgent warnings that something is wrong. This shift is subtle but impactful: people stop planning their lives around pain, movement becomes easier, and trust replaces constant vigilance. Importantly, this doesn't require constant effort. Once the nervous system learns to calm down, regulation becomes a skill that works in the background.

Pain relief usually isn't about fixing a single issue; it's about restoring balance to systems under prolonged strain. You've learned how stress affects pain, how awareness creates choice, how tension can ease, and how movement helps the body adapt, how strength builds confidence, and how regulation allows everything to settle.[16]

Progress isn't always linear. Some days may feel harder, but that doesn't mean you've lost ground; it reflects how your system responds to life. The aim isn't to eliminate all sensation, but to build a body and nervous system that are strong, adaptable, and safe enough to move through life without constant guard. That is what lasting relief truly means. This isn't the end; it's the beginning of living with more freedom.

CHAPTER 7

Integrating It All: Your Pain-Free Daily System

Small daily movement beats occasional big effort—every time.

Creating a pain-free life does not happen overnight. It requires consistent, small efforts rather than sporadic, intense bursts of activity. In this chapter, we'll explore how to integrate effective movement, relaxation, and strength-building into your daily routine. By establishing a sustainable system, you can alleviate stress, reduce pain, and enhance your overall quality of life. Most pain programs fail for one simple reason: they don't survive real life. People often begin their journeys with strong motivation. They diligently follow their plans, carve out time for their goals, and initially experience improvement. However, as work and life become busier, stress levels rise, sleep suffers, and symptoms may resurface. This disruption can break their routine and bring back pain. As a result, many may feel a discouraging conclusion: that their efforts never truly stick.

But the problem is rarely the person. It's the structure.

Long-term pain relief doesn't depend only on motivation or strict discipline. It relies on systems that can handle stress without breaking down. These systems fit into your life, rather than working against it, and keep going even when motivation fades.

This chapter will show you how to build that system.

By now, you have all the parts: calming your nervous system, becoming more aware, letting go of tension, moving better, building strength safely, and managing stress. The next step is to learn how to integrate these into your daily routine, so they support you with minimal effort. This isn't about doing more. It's about doing just enough, regularly, to keep things balanced.

How to Build a Sustainable Routine

Most routines don't last because they depend on effort instead of identity. When people say, "I need to be more consistent," they usually mean, "I need to push myself harder." But real consistency doesn't come from forcing yourself. It comes from matching your actions with how you see yourself.

Habits based on identity work because they shift your focus. Instead of asking, Did I do my exercises today? You start to ask, what would someone who takes care of their body do right now?

This shift is subtle but powerful.

People who stick with routines for a long time don't treat movement as a chore. They see it as part of their identity. Like brushing your teeth or making coffee, it just happens without much thought. At first, you do need some discipline. Whether it's exercise, work, business, or health, you build consistency before it feels automatic. Discipline helps you keep going until the habit sticks.

Behavior stacking makes this process easier. Rather than blocking out large amounts of time, you add small practices to your existing habits. For example, take a few deep breaths after you stand up, move a bit before sitting down, or take a quick break after work. These actions are so simple that you're likely to stick with them, and that's what makes them effective.

Over time, having a steady routine becomes more important than relying on discipline. Discipline means using willpower, while rhythm comes from repeating actions. When you move and regulate yourself at about the same times each day, your nervous system starts to expect it. This regularity can help lower your overall tension. This is especially helpful for managing pain. When your body expects relief, it doesn't react as strongly while waiting for it.

Behavior Stacking

Behavior stacking involves linking a new habit to an existing one, making it easier to incorporate into your daily life. For example, if you already have a morning coffee ritual, add a five-minute stretching routine immediately after. This makes it more likely you'll stick to the new behavior, as it becomes part of an established routine.

One example of habit stacking could be changing a current habit, such as drinking coffee. Instead of simply enjoying the coffee, you could introduce a new habit of doing five minutes of stretching. This would create a stacked routine where you say to yourself, "After I finish my coffee, I will do five minutes of stretching." This approach not only helps in maintaining the pleasurable routine of coffee drinking but also integrates a healthy practice into your day.

Choose Rhythm Over Strict Discipline

Instead of relying solely on willpower, focus on establishing a steady routine that allows for a natural flow throughout your day. Set specific times for movement, relaxation, and strength training, but make sure to include flexibility for when life gets busy.

Start your morning with mobility exercises to help you ease into the day. Around midday, take a short break to give yourself a quick reset. In the evening, unwind with some gentle stretching or yoga.

By creating a consistent rhythm, you'll find it easier to incorporate movement into your day without the added stress. This approach not only supports your physical well-being but also enhances your overall balance and productivity.

Real-World Example

One client struggled for years to maintain an exercise routine, consistently experiencing initial motivation followed by burnout. By limiting movement to three brief daily sessions (morning, midday, and evening), it became a regular part of the day rather than an option. Pain improved because resistance disappeared, not due to increased effort.

The Minimum Effective Dose

Building a sustainable routine means making small changes that fit into your everyday life. The minimum effective dose is the smallest amount of effort required to produce results. This will, however, look different for each person, depending on their current condition, energy levels, and daily demands. As a general starting point, many people benefit from aiming for around 25-30 minutes of movement per day, combined with regular walking.

For most people dealing with pain, this means:

- 5 to 10 minutes of movement in the morning
- 2 to 3 brief resets during the day (1 to 2 minutes each)
- 5 to 10 minutes of gentle evening practice

That's it. Total time: 15 to 25 minutes spread across the entire day. Research supports this approach. Studies show that movement frequency, not duration, matters more for reducing chronic pain. Small, repeated doses of regulation help the nervous system stay balanced better than occasional long sessions.

The goal is not to maximize effort. It's to maintain consistency without burnout. When you keep the bar low, you're more likely to clear it every day. And daily consistency is what changes your nervous system's baseline.

Even just five minutes a day can be more effective than thirty minutes once in a while. Short, regular practice lowers pressure and helps you avoid all-or-nothing thinking, which can lead to setbacks. As you get more consistent, you can add more time if you want, but you should never feel like you have to.

The Stress-Pain Relief Daily Flow

Instead of focusing on workouts, think of your day as a flow. Your day already has its own rhythm, and pain relief is most effective when it follows that natural pattern. A basic daily flow includes three parts: morning, midday, and evening. Each part plays a unique role and supports your nervous system in its own way.

Morning: Setting the Baseline

The morning sets the tone for your day. After sleeping, your body may feel stiff, and your nervous system can be a bit on edge. Instead of stretching hard or trying to wake up quickly, focus on gentle movements that help you loosen up and ease early tension. Gentle mobility is best in the morning. Try slow neck and spine movements, and gentle hip circles. Keep everything relaxed and unhurried. Your breathing should stay calm and easy. If it gets short, ease up on the movement.

This gentle start signals to your nervous system that the day is safe. Over time, this can help reduce morning pain.

Example Morning Sequence (5 minutes)

- Gentle neck rotations within a comfortable range
- Rib expansion with slow breathing
- Hip mobility in standing or on the floor

Remember, this is gentle preparation for the day ahead.

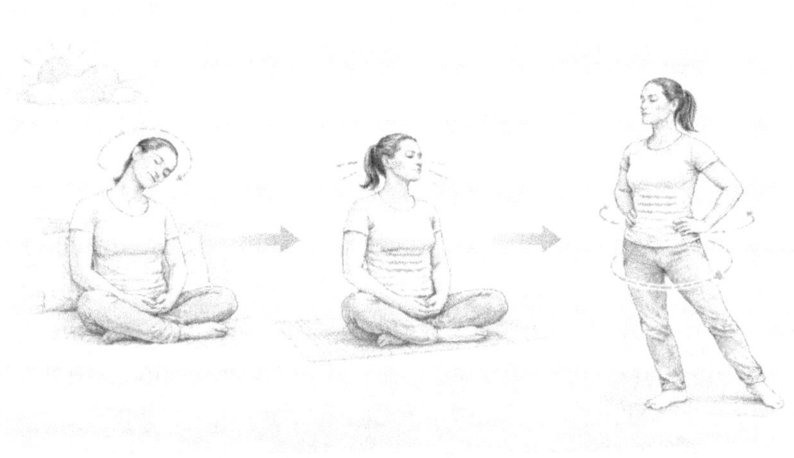

Figure 7.1: Morning flow

Midday: Breaking Up Built-Up Tension

Around midday, pain often builds up. Sitting for long periods, focusing, and dealing with stress can slowly make your muscles tense and sensitive. Pain often only becomes noticeable once your body is already irritated, so the goal is to break this cycle. Even a minute-long break, standing, shifting your weight, or taking a few slow breaths, can help prevent tension from building.

Try standing up, shifting your position, taking a few slow breaths, or letting your eyes rest. Your nervous system likes new, gentle actions. These midday habits should be simple to add to your day, not feel like extra work.

Example Midday Reset (1 to 2 minutes)

- Stand up and shift your weight side to side
- Roll the shoulders slowly
- Take three slow breaths with longer exhales
- Do some spine movements

Done once or twice, this can prevent evening flare-ups.

Evening: Helping Your Body Unwind

Many people notice pain most in the evening. Once the day's demands end, your body finally has a chance to feel what it's been holding. Without a conscious effort to relax, your system can stay tense into the night, making it harder to sleep and recover. Evening routines should help you feel calm, not like you need to fix something. Gentle movement, slower breathing, and less stimulation signal to your body that it's safe to rest. This step isn't about improving your posture or increasing flexibility. It's simply about letting go of tension.

Example Evening Wind-Down (5 to 10 minutes)

- Floor-based positions or gentle stretching
- Slow breathing with longer exhales
- 60-second attention reset

Consistency matters more than duration.

Why This Flow Works

This daily routine helps avoid extremes. Rather than working too hard and then burning out, you stay within comfortable limits. Pain sensitivity stays lower since tension does not have time to build up. With time, this routine becomes second nature. Your body starts to expect movement, rest, and balance at certain times each day. Just having that routine helps reduce tension and guarding.

Weekly Strength and Movement Plan

Moving every day helps keep your nervous system calm, and having a weekly routine builds physical confidence. Both matter. Many people try to do every activity every day, but this can feel overwhelming. If you make mobility, strength, release work, breathing, walking, and posture resets daily tasks, it adds extra stress. We want to make things easier. A weekly plan gives you flexibility, allowing some lighter days and some heavier ones. This approach aligns with real life and helps your body adjust rather than getting tense.

The purpose of a weekly plan is to find balance, not to do as much as possible. Strength and mobility support each other. Mobility keeps options available. Strength allows those options to feel safe under load. Neither needs to dominate the week.

Anchor Days: The Essentials You Commit To

Anchor days help you build a sustainable week. On these days, you set aside a bit more time for movement, no matter how busy you are. The sessions don't need to be intense; they just need to be consistent. For most people, two to three anchor days work well. On anchor days, focus on strength exercises. Practice push, pull, hinge, and squat movements, paying attention to your breath and control. You can add mobility work to your warm-up or cool-down, but the main goal is to build strength and ability. Anchor days create continuity. Even if the rest of the week is unpredictable, these days remind the system that strength and movement are part of life.

Sample Anchor Day Routine (20 to 30 minutes)

- **5 minutes:** gentle mobility and breathing
- **10 to 20 minutes:** strength movement patterns (pick 5 exercises from Chapter 5)
- **5 minutes:** slow down and recover

You don't need to feel worn out after this. The goal is to feel steady and grounded.

Flexible Days: Focus on Support, Not Competition

Keep the rest of the week flexible. Use these days for lighter activities like walking, mobility work, or recovery. If you feel stressed or low on energy, it's often better to take it easy. Flexible days help you avoid the all-or-nothing mindset. They let you stay active without making movement feel like a chore.

On flexible days, try short routines from earlier chapters. Gentle stretches, alignment exercises, or calming movements with focused breathing can help you feel safe and supported.

Real-World Example

One client found it hard to keep up with a five-day training schedule. When they switched to two anchor days and three flexible sessions, they stuck with it better and felt less pain because the routine was easier to manage. This doesn't mean you should avoid training often or pushing yourself. I often train hard, but for someone just starting, gentle consistency matters most. High volume and intensity can be good and even fun when your body is ready for it.

Timing is crucial. If you are recovering and experiencing pain, poor sleep, or high stress, increasing intensity may add unnecessary pressure. Beginning with a gentle approach is not a weakness. It prepares you for more challenging training later.

Walking as a Consistent Weekly Practice

Walking has a lot of benefits. It improves circulation, coordination, breathing, and helps you manage emotions. No preparation is needed. You can walk even on low-energy days. If formal exercise feels difficult, regular walks can help reduce pain. The steady pace is also good for your nervous system. For many people, walking is a habit they can count on each week.

This weekly approach is not about perfection. Some weeks will go as planned, others won't. What matters is that you keep returning to the structure without judgment. Anchor days give you direction. Flexible days give you space. Together, they create a system you can actually live with.

Measuring Progress (Without Pain Obsession)

Pain is not a reliable indicator of progress, as it can fluctuate for various reasons that don't necessarily reflect improvements. Focusing solely on pain can heighten anxiety and caution, which may, in turn, exacerbate the pain. To track your progress more effectively, it's essential to look beyond just pain levels. Consider how easily you can get out of a chair, the effort required to walk, and how quickly you recover after activities. Often, these improvements manifest before any pain reduction is felt.

Emotional changes also play a significant role in progress. Feeling less frustrated, worrying less about movement, being more willing to engage in physical activities, and gaining confidence are all positive indicators. A key sign of progress is no longer asking yourself, "Will this hurt?" before doing things.

You don't need to document every detail of your journey; simply reflecting on your week can suffice. Ask yourself:

- Do daily tasks feel more manageable?
- Do flare-ups settle faster than they used to?
- Am I thinking about my body less often?
- Does movement feel less risky?

If your answers to these questions begin to shift, it means you are making real progress.

Letting Go of the Pain Score

Numeric pain scales can help at first, but over time, they may hold people back. Instead of aiming for better movement, people start to focus only on getting a lower pain score. This keeps attention on symptoms rather than on what the body can do. As you make progress, it can help to stop rating your pain and start paying attention to what your body can do. In most cases, pain eases as your function improves, not the other way around.

Action Steps: The 7-Day Jumpstart Program

This program helps you get started gently. It aims to help you feel more connected, not to test your skills. Each day, you'll do a bit more. If something feels like too much, try it for a shorter time instead of skipping it.

Day 1: Set Your Starting Point

- **Morning:** Spend 5 to 10 minutes moving gently (for example, neck movements, downward facing dog, cat-cow movements)
- **Midday:** One 60-second reset, ankle pumps, thoracic rotations
- **Evening:** Practice slow breathing for 3 to 5 minutes (for example, box breathing)

Pay attention to how your body feels, without trying to change anything.

Day 2: Try Different Types of Movement

- **Morning:** Move your neck, ribs, and hips (choose 3 exercises from earlier book chapters)
- **Midday:** Short walk or a reminder to change posture during the day (especially important for desk workers)
- **Evening:** Gentle floor-based movement (for example, supine pelvic tilt sequence, supine twist, hip and knee sequence on the floor)

The goal is variety, not intensity.

Day 3: Start Strength Training with a Gentle Approach

Strength session (10 to 15 minutes):

- Do one push exercise for 10 to 30 repetitions (for example, wall push-up, push-up)
- Do one pull exercise for 10 to 30 repetitions (for example, pull-up, dumbbell row)
- Do one hinge exercise for 10 to 30 repetitions (for example, single-leg hinge)

- Do one squat exercise for 10 to 30 repetitions (for example, wall-sit, loaded squat)

Remember to keep your breathing steady and stop before you feel tired. Start at the lower end of the range and increase only if it feels comfortable.

Day 4: Focus on Recovery and Regulation

To promote overall well-being, consider incorporating gentle activities into your routine, such as taking a walk or engaging in a slow run. Additionally, exploring breath-led movement can enhance your physical awareness and relaxation. Be sure to dedicate extra time winding down in the evening, allowing your body and mind to transition into a restful state.

Throughout this process, pay close attention to how these practices influence your recovery, pain levels, and energy throughout the day.

Day 5: Strength Anchor Day

To achieve a well-rounded fitness routine, make sure to complete the full-strength exercises outlined in Chapter 5, which include push, pull, hinge, and squat movements. After your workout, take the time to cool down and allow your body to recover. Always remember that feeling confident in your abilities is more important than pushing yourself too hard. Prioritize your well-being and listen to your body as you progress.

Day 6: Flexible Movement

Pick what feels best for you today, whether that's walking, gentle movement, stretching, or simply taking a break.

Any option you choose is the right one for you.

Day 7: Take Time to Reflect and Make Changes

Start with a quick reflection:

- What was helpful for you?
- What did you find unnecessary?
- What do you think you can keep doing long-term?

Let your answers guide how you plan for the week ahead.

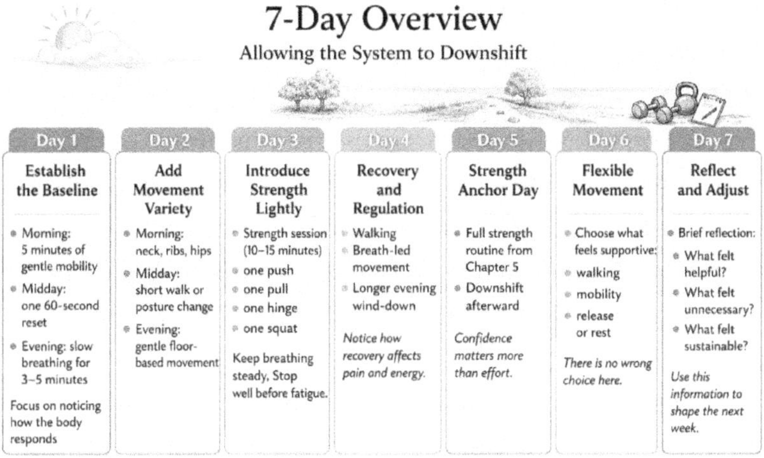

Figure 7.2: 7-day overview calendar

Final Thoughts

These practices offer consistent relief. Living without pain does not require perfect days; it requires adaptable systems for challenging times. Regular small movements help retrain your nervous system. Over time, you will feel calmer and more confident. You no longer need to seek quick fixes, as you now have a supportive structure in place. Your body does not require strict control. Instead, listen to it, offer support, and let it respond naturally. This approach helps movement become a natural part of your life, rather than an added task.

A Reflection

Consistency is often mistaken for simply repeating actions. In reality, identity is the true foundation of consistent behavior. People struggle with consistency because their actions do not align with who they believe they are, not because they forget what to do. When behavior and identity are aligned, consistency occurs naturally. When they are not, it feels forced. This is why true consistency is not built through reminders, motivation, or pressure, but through identity.

Consistency is not about pushing harder. It is about becoming someone whose behavior makes sense. To achieve long-term consistency, focus on your actions and on who you need to become.

Until identity is defined, behavior will always drift. Discipline will come and go. Progress will stay inconsistent. When identity and behavior align, sustainable growth is possible in daily exercise and in other areas.

Consider the following:
Rather than asking, "How can I stay consistent with exercise when I am in pain?" it is more beneficial to ask, "Whom do I need to become for this behavior to feel natural?" This shift in perspective encourages personal growth and the development of a mindset that aligns with the desired behavior.

CONCLUSION:

The New You–Stronger, Calmer, and Pain-Free

For many, the hardest part of living with pain isn't the feeling itself, but what it seems to say about them. Pain is often seen as proof that something is wrong, that the body has failed, or that past choices can't be undone. Over time, this belief can feel heavier than the pain itself. But pain is not a judgment of your worth or discipline. It is information. Your body responds to the conditions it faces: stress that lasts too long, movement that becomes limited or repetitive, rest that doesn't fully restore, and emotional pressure with no outlet. Pain shows up as a signal that your system is overloaded and trying its best to cope.

When you see pain this way, the story changes. Instead of asking, "What is wrong with me?" you might ask, "What has my body been managing for a long time without enough support?" This shift removes blame and makes change possible.

This book isn't about getting rid of symptoms as fast as possible. It's about learning to listen to the message behind them. When that message is clearer, pain no longer feels random or threatening. It becomes something you can respond to instead of fear.

Why Nothing Was Ever "Broken"

As a physiotherapist, I often meet people who have been told their bodies are worn out, misaligned, or beyond repair.

These messages can be hard to shake, especially when they come with medical images or medical language that sounds final. Over time, these beliefs can affect how people move, breathe, and even how they see their future. But in my experience, things often look different. Some people have major changes on their scans, but move easily and feel fine. Others have only minor changes but deal with pain every day. Anatomy alone usually does not explain these differences.

The human body is always adapting to what it goes through. If movement feels unsafe, muscles tighten up. If stress stays high, the body becomes more sensitive. If sleep is poor, recovery takes longer. This does not mean the body is broken. It means it is doing what it is meant to do.

As the nervous system feels safer, those reactions begin to calm down. Muscles loosen up, movement becomes easier, and sensations become less intense. This change occurs because the body no longer has to protect itself as much, not because something was repaired. Pain often goes away once we feel safe again.

From Control to Cooperation

Many people begin their healing process by trying to control their bodies. They search for the right exercises, the correct posture, and the perfect routine. When pain is unpredictable, control seems like the logical answer. It offers a sense of stability.

But the body does not respond well to control alone. It responds better to cooperation. In this book, you were encouraged to stop forcing change and instead create the right conditions for change to happen naturally. Rather than tightening more, you learned to let go. Rather than pushing through fear, you learned to work with it. Rather than correcting every movement, you learned to bring back more options.

This approach takes patience, but it helps you build trust. Trust can make a big difference. When your body trusts that movement will not lead to pain, it allows more freedom. When your nervous system trusts that stress will be handled with care rather than ignored, it calms down more quickly. Over time, this cooperation becomes natural. You stop micromanaging your body and start listening to it.

Strength That Feels Supportive

As an athlete, I learned early that strength without awareness leads to injury. If you push through tiredness, ignore warning signs, or see rest as a weakness, it eventually takes a toll. The same idea applies to healing.

Strength helps most when it feels supportive rather than demanding. You've learned how to build strength in ways that respect your nervous system. Strength that works with breath. Strength that allows movement to stay smooth. Strength that prepares you for life rather than testing your limits. This kind of strength stays with you, even when life gets stressful. It acts as a buffer, making daily tasks easier, helping you handle surprises, and speeding up your recovery. Strength stops being just an action and becomes something you can count on.

Calm Is a Skill, Not a Personality Trait

Many people think you are either born calm or not, and that it depends on your personality or mindset. In fact, calm is a state your body can learn through practice. You have learned to calm your nervous system by using your breath, moving your body, and focusing your attention. These methods do not eliminate emotions or stress, but they help keep you from feeling overwhelmed.

Being calm does not mean you are never affected by things. It means you can bounce back more quickly. This difference is important. A body that can settle down after stress is much stronger than one that never reacts. Regulation is about being flexible, not about controlling everything. With practice, calm starts to feel normal. Your body gets used to it and returns to it faster. Pain also feels less intense because it is not fighting against constant tension.

Becoming Someone Who Trusts Their Body

The most important change might not be physical. It's about connecting with your body. When pain shows up, trust can fade fast. Movements seem risky. Sensations feel strange. As you go through this process, trust returns slowly. You figure out which feelings are safe to move through. You learn to adjust rather than avoid things. You also realize that discomfort doesn't always mean something is wrong. You build this trust through experience, not just by being reassured. Each calm repetition helps. Each time pain flares up, it settles a bit faster than before. Day by day, moving feels less like a struggle. In time, you stop waiting for your body's permission to live and start including it in your life.

What "Pain-Free" Really Means

Being pain-free does not mean you will never feel discomfort again. Our bodies are alive, and feeling things is a natural part of life.

Pain-free means pain is no longer in control of your life.

You start making choices based on what matters to you, not just your symptoms. You move more freely, rest without worrying about setbacks, and trust your body to handle what comes. This is a deeper form of relief. One that lasts because it is rooted in adaptability rather than avoidance.

A hopeful truth about the human body is that it can adapt no matter how much time has passed. Even after years of pain, setbacks, or inactivity, this ability does not go away. It might slow down and need more patience, but it is always there. I have worked with people who thought they were too old, too stiff, or beyond help. Many had already tried everything they knew. What helped them was a new way of relating to their body, not a new method. When they felt less fear and focused on being consistent rather than rushing, they began to see change.

The body adapts when it gets clear, repeated signals that it is safe to change. This happens when you move in different ways, build strength slowly, and handle stress by calming yourself instead of pushing it down. These signals let your nervous system know it can relax its guard. This process does not demand perfection. What matters is being present and patient. This opportunity is open to you at any age.

Movement Is a Lifelong Companion

Movement isn't something you finish or leave behind. It's always part of life as long as you're in your body. Sometimes, moving feels easy and expressive. Other times, it's quieter and more about getting things done. Some periods are challenging, while others need a gentler touch. Every stage is important. When you think of movement as a lifelong companion rather than a task, it stops feeling like something you start and then stop. It becomes something that grows with you. This is how pain relief can last. Moving helps your blood flow, keeps your joints working, and keeps your nervous system focused on the present. It also helps prevent stress from building up and gives your emotions a way out.

As a physiotherapist, athlete, and yoga teacher, I have seen that regular, flexible movement helps people feel better. The goal is not to do more, but to move in ways that feel right for you. When you move and focus on your breath, you create space in your body and mind, so you can notice sensations without feeling overwhelmed. From my experience, movement works best when practiced with awareness and respect.

Carrying This Work Forward

Over time, these steps become automatic. Instead of thinking through each one, you begin to respond naturally. You notice stress earlier, move instead of freezing, and adjust calmly when pain shows up. That's integration.

Even so, symptoms may still return at times. This doesn't mean you've lost progress. It usually means your body needs something different. The difference now is that you can respond without panic—whether that's rest, movement, or breath. You're not starting from scratch.

As this continues, your identity can begin to shift. You may catch yourself moving more freely or thinking about your body less. These are signs of progress. Your past is still part of you, but it no longer has to shape every decision.

At a deeper level, resilience is the ability to shift between effort and rest. You've built strength without excess tension and learned to stay calm under stress. As a result, everyday movement feels easier, and pain becomes less urgent.

A Personal Reflection

Writing this book comes from years of listening to patients, friends, and my own body. Whether in physiotherapy clinics, yoga studios, or at the climbing wall, I keep seeing the same patterns. People heal when they feel safe enough to change.

Safety doesn't come from following rules. It grows from being consistent, staying curious, and respecting what the body tells us. It also comes from learning to respond rather than just react.

If you remember just one thing from this book, let it be that your body has always been on your side. Even when you felt pain, confusion, or slow progress, your body was not broken. Pain simply meant something needed attention. Now, you have what you need to give that care. You may not do it perfectly or all the time, but you can do it often enough to see real change.

You are stronger than you were. Calmer than you were. More capable than you were taught to believe.

And that strength will continue to grow as long as you keep listening to your body.

This is not an ending. It is a steadier beginning.

Author's Request

Dear Reader,

If this book helped you understand your pain differently, feel safer in your body, or move with more confidence, I'd be deeply grateful if you shared your experience.

Leaving a short review helps others who are feeling lost, frustrated, or unsure where to turn realize that change is possible. You don't need to write anything long or perfect—just a few honest words about what this book gave you, or how it supported you, is enough.

Your review helps this work reach the people who need it most.

If you found this book helpful, I would truly appreciate you taking a moment to share your experience with a review on Amazon.

Thank you for taking the time to read, reflect, and care for your body.

With gratitude,
Tina

Notes & References

Introduction

[1] Inge Timmers et al. "The interaction between stress and chronic pain through the lens of threat learning", *Neuroscience & Biobehavioral Reviews* 107, nº 1 (décembre 2019): 641-55. https://doi.org/10.1016/j.neubiorev.2019.10.007.
[2] G. Lorimer Moseley et David S. Butler. "Fifteen Years of Explaining Pain: The Past, Present, and Future", *The Journal of Pain* 16, nº 9 (septembre 2015): 807-13. https://doi.org/10.1016/j.jpain.2015.05.005.
[3] Timmers et al., "Interaction Between Stress and Chronic Pain," 643.
[4] Bessel van der Kolk, *The body keeps the score: brain, mind and body in the healing of trauma* (New York: Penguin Books, 2015).
[5] Temitayo Olugbade, Nadia Bianchi-Berthouze, et Amanda C de C. Williams. "The relationship between guarding, pain, and emotion", *PAIN Reports* 4, nº 4 (2019): e770. https://www.ncbi.nlm.nih.gov/pmc/articles/PMC6728010/.
[6] Emma Meehan et Bernie Carter. "Moving With Pain: What Principles From Somatic Practices Can Offer to People Living with Chronic Pain", *Frontiers in Psychology* 11 (25 janvier 2021). https://doi.org/10.3389/fpsyg.2020.620381.

Chapter 1

[1] Chou R, Qaseem A, Snow V, Casey D, Cross JT Jr, Shekelle P, Owens DK. *Diagnosis and treatment of low back pain: a joint clinical practice guideline from the American College of Physicians and the American Pain Society.* Annals of Internal Medicine. 2007;147(7):478–491. doi:10.7326/0003-4819-147-7-200710020-00006.
[2] International Association for the Study of Pain. *Terminology,* International Association for the Study of Pain (IASP), 2020. https://www.iasp-pain.org/resources/terminology/.
[3] Emily L Zale et Joseph W Ditre. "Pain-related fear, disability, and the fear-avoidance model of chronic pain", *Current Opinion in Psychology* 5, nº 5 (octobre 2015): 24-30. https://doi.org/10.1016/j.copsyc.2015.03.014.

[4] Dirk De Ridder, Divya Adhia, et Sven Vanneste. "The Anatomy of Pain and Suffering in the Brain and Its Clinical Implications", *Neuroscience & Biobehavioral Reviews* 130, n° 130 (novembre 2021): 125-46. https://doi.org/10.1016/j.neubiorev.2021.08.013.

[5] Brianna Chu et al., "Physiology, Stress Reaction," PubMed (Treasure Island (FL): StatPearls Publishing, May 7, 2024), https://www.ncbi.nlm.nih.gov/books/NBK541120/.

[6] Gabor Maté, MD, *When the Body Says No* (Vintage Canada, 2011).

[7] Dalius Bansevicius, Rolf H. Westgaard, and Chris Jensen, "Mental Stress of Long Duration: EMG Activity, Perceived Tension, Fatigue, and Pain Development in Pain-Free Subjects," Headache 37, no. 8 (1997): 499–510, https://doi.org/10.1046/j.1526-4610.1997.3708499.x.

[8] Bessel van der Kolk, *The body keeps the score: brain, mind and body in the healing of trauma* (New York: Penguin Books, 2015).

[9] G. Lorimer Moseley and David S. Butler, "Fifteen Years of Explaining Pain: The Past, Present, and Future," *The Journal of Pain* 16, no. 9 (September 2015): 807–13, https://doi.org/10.1016/j.jpain.2015.05.005.

[10] Moseley and Butler, "Fifteen Years of Explaining Pain," 809; K. Wiech, "Deconstructing the Sensation of Pain: The Influence of Cognitive Processes on Pain Perception," *Science* 354, no. 6312 (November 3, 2016): 584–87, https://doi.org/10.1126/science.aaf8934.

[11] Johan W.S. Vlaeyen and Steven J. Linton, "Fear-Avoidance and Its Consequences in Chronic Musculoskeletal Pain: A State of the Art," *Pain* 85, no. 3 (April 2000): 317–32, https://doi.org/10.1016/s0304-3959(99)00242-0; Zale and Ditre, "Pain-Related Fear," 26.

[12] Paul R. Martin, "Behavioral Management of Migraine Headache Triggers: Learning to Cope with Triggers," *Current Pain and Headache Reports* 14, no. 3 (April 27, 2010): 221–27, https://doi.org/10.1007/s11916-010-0112-z.

[13] Timmers, I., et al. "Brain Mechanisms of Expectation in Pain." *Journal of Neuroscience* 39, no. 14 (2019): 2553–2565.; K. Wiech, "Deconstructing the Sensation of Pain: The Influence of Cognitive Processes on Pain Perception," *Science* 354, no. 6312 (November 3, 2016): 584–87, https://doi.org/10.1126/science.aaf8934.

[14] Moseley and Butler, "Fifteen Years of Explaining Pain," 809 ; Adriaan Louw et al., "The Efficacy of Pain Neuroscience Education on Musculoskeletal Pain: A Systematic Review of the Literature,"

Physiotherapy Theory and Practice 32, no. 5 (June 28, 2016): 332–55, https://doi.org/10.1080/09593985.2016.1194646.

[15] Matthew A. Stults-Kolehmainen, "Humans Have a Basic Physical and Psychological Need to Move the Body: Physical Activity as a Primary Drive," *Frontiers in Psychology* 14 (April 11, 2023), https://doi.org/10.3389/fpsyg.2023.1134049.

[16] Frank W. Booth, Christian K. Roberts, and Matthew J. Laye, "Lack of Exercise Is a Major Cause of Chronic Diseases," *Comprehensive Physiology* 2, no. 2 (April 2012), https://doi.org/10.1002/cphy.c110025.

[17] Eugene G. McNally, et al., "Joint Lubrication and the Role of Synovial Fluid," *Radiologic Clinics of North America* 40, no. 5 (2002): 1117–1132; W.B. van den Berg, "Osteoarthritis Year 2010 in Review: Pathomechanisms," *Osteoarthritis and Cartilage* 19, no. 4 (April 2011): 338–41, https://doi.org/10.1016/j.joca.2011.01.022.

[18] Aviroop Biswas et al., "Sedentary Time and Its Association with Risk for Disease Incidence, Mortality, and Hospitalization in Adults," *Annals of Internal Medicine* 162, no. 2 (January 20, 2015): 123, https://doi.org/10.7326/m14-1651; Jason A Bennie et al., "The Prevalence and Correlates of Sitting in European Adults - a Comparison of 32 Eurobarometer-Participating Countries," *International Journal of Behavioral Nutrition and Physical Activity* 10, no. 1 (2013): 107, https://doi.org/10.1186/1479-5868-10-107.

[19] Rayane Haddadj et al., "Volume and Intensity of Walking and Risk of Chronic Low Back Pain," *JAMA Network Open* 8, no. 6 (June 13, 2025): e2515592–92, https://doi.org/10.1001/jamanetworkopen.2025.15592.

[20] R. Shiri and K. Falah-Hassani, "Does Leisure Time Physical Activity Protect Against Low Back Pain? Systematic Review and Meta-Analysis of 36 Prospective Cohort Studies," *British Journal of Sports Medicine* 51, no. 19 (2017): 1410–1418, https://doi.org/10.1136/bjsports-2016-097352..

[21] Vlaeyen and Linton, "Fear-Avoidance and Its Consequences," 320; Olugbade, Bianchi-Berthouze, and Williams, "The Relationship between Guarding, Pain, and Emotion."

[22] Woolf, "Central Sensitization," S10; Moseley and Butler, "Fifteen Years of Explaining Pain," 809.

[23] A. Vania Apkarian, Marwan N. Baliki, and Paul Y. Geha, "Towards a Theory of Chronic Pain," *Progress in Neurobiology* 87, no. 2 (February 2009): 81–97, https://doi.org/10.1016/j.pneurobio.2008.09.018; G.

Lorimer Moseley and Herta Flor, "Targeting Cortical Representations in the Treatment of Chronic Pain," *Neurorehabilitation and Neural Repair* 26, no. 6 (February 13, 2012): 646–52, https://doi.org/10.1177/1545968311433209.
[24] Woolf, "Central Sensitization," S10.
[25] Patrick H. Finan, Burel R. Goodin, and Michael T. Smith, "The Association of Sleep and Pain: An Update and a Path Forward," *The Journal of Pain* 14, no. 12 (December 2013): 1539–52, https://doi.org/10.1016/j.jpain.2013.08.007.
[26] Cynthia Holzman Weppler and S. Peter Magnusson, "Increasing Muscle Extensibility: A Matter of Increasing Length or Modifying Sensation?" *Physical Therapy* 90, no. 3 (2010): 438–449, https://doi.org/10.2522/ptj.20090012; Apostolos Apostolopoulos et al., "The Relevance of Stretch Intensity and Position—A Systematic Review," *Frontiers in Psychology* 6 (2015): 1128, https://doi.org/10.3389/fpsyg.2015.01128..
[27] Meehan and Carter, "Moving with Pain."
[28] Paul W. Hodges and G.Lorimer Moseley, "Pain and Motor Control of the Lumbopelvic Region: Effect and Possible Mechanisms," *Journal of Electromyography and Kinesiology* 13, no. 4 (August 2003): 361–70, https://doi.org/10.1016/s1050-6411(03)00042-7.
[29] Finan, Goodin, and Smith, "The Association of Sleep and Pain," 1545.
[30] Apkarian, Baliki, and Geha, "Towards a Theory of Chronic Pain," 85; Moseley and Flor, "Targeting Cortical Representations," 648.
[31] Sara Magelssen Vambheim et al., "Relaxation Techniques as an Intervention for Chronic Pain: A Systematic Review of Randomized Controlled Trials," *Heliyon* 7, no. 8 (August 2021): e07837, https://doi.org/10.1016/j.heliyon.2021.e07837.
[32] Moseley and Butler, "Fifteen Years of Explaining Pain," 809.
[33] Ulf Lundberg et al., "Psychophysiological Stress and Emg Activity of the Trapezius Muscle," *International Journal of Behavioral Medicine* 1, no. 4 (December 1994): 354–70, https://doi.org/10.1207/s15327558ijbm0104_5.
[34] Julia Treleaven, "Sensorimotor Disturbances in Neck Disorders Affecting Postural Stability, Head and Eye Movement Control," *Manual Therapy* 13, no. 1 (February 2008): 2–11, https://doi.org/10.1016/j.math.2007.06.003.

Chapter 2

[1] Bessel van der Kolk, *The Body Keeps the Score: Brain, Mind and Body in the Healing of Trauma* (New York: Penguin Books, 2015).
[2] Jason A Bennie et al., "The Prevalence and Correlates of Sitting in European Adults - a Comparison of 32 Eurobarometer-Participating Countries," *International Journal of Behavioral Nutrition and Physical Activity* 10, no. 1 (2013): 107, https://doi.org/10.1186/1479-5868-10-107.
[3] P.-P.A. Vergroesen et al., "Mechanics and Biology in Intervertebral Disc Degeneration: A Vicious Circle," *Osteoarthritis and Cartilage* 23, no. 7 (July 2015): 1057–70, https://doi.org/10.1016/j.joca.2015.03.028.
[4] P E Williams and G Goldspink, "Connective Tissue Changes in Immobilised Muscle," *Journal of Anatomy* 138, no. Pt 2 (March 1984): 343, https://pmc.ncbi.nlm.nih.gov/articles/PMC1164074/.
[5] G. Lorimer Moseley and Herta Flor, "Targeting Cortical Representations in the Treatment of Chronic Pain," *Neurorehabilitation and Neural Repair* 26, no. 6 (February 13, 2012): 646–52, https://doi.org/10.1177/1545968311433209; Herta Flor et al., "Extensive Reorganization of Primary Somatosensory Cortex in Chronic Back Pain Patients," *Neuroscience Letters* 224, no. 1 (March 1997): 5–8, https://doi.org/10.1016/s0304-3940(97)13441-3.
[6] G. Lorimer Moseley and David S. Butler, "Fifteen Years of Explaining Pain: The Past, Present, and Future," *The Journal of Pain* 16, no. 9 (September 2015): 807–13, https://doi.org/10.1016/j.jpain.2015.05.005.
[7] A. D. Craig, "How Do You Feel? Interoception: The Sense of the Physiological Condition of the Body," *Nature Reviews Neuroscience* 3, no. 8 (August 2002): 655–66, https://doi.org/10.1038/nrn894; Wolf E. Mehling et al., "The Multidimensional Assessment of Interoceptive Awareness (MAIA)," ed. Manos Tsakiris, *PLoS ONE* 7, no. 11 (November 1, 2012): e48230, https://doi.org/10.1371/journal.pone.0048230.
[8] Flor et al., "Extensive Reorganization of Primary Somatosensory Cortex in Chronic Back Pain Patients."; Moseley and Flor, "Targeting Cortical Representations in the Treatment of Chronic Pain."
[9]G.L Moseley, "A Pain Neuromatrix Approach to Patients with Chronic Pain," *Manual Therapy* 8, no. 3 (August 2003): 130–40, https://doi.org/10.1016/s1356-689x(03)00051-1.
[10] Moseley and Butler, "Fifteen Years of Explaining Pain."

[11] Eric L. Garland et al., "Mindfulness-Oriented Recovery Enhancement Reduces Opioid Dose in Primary Care by Strengthening Autonomic Regulation during Meditation.," *American Psychologist* 75, no. 6 (September 2020): 840–52, https://doi.org/10.1037/amp0000638; F. Zeidan et al., "Mindfulness Meditation-Related Pain Relief: Evidence for Unique Brain Mechanisms in the Regulation of Pain," *Neuroscience Letters* 520, no. 2 (June 2012): 165–73,
https://doi.org/10.1016/j.neulet.2012.03.082.
[12] Ulf Lundberg et al., "Psychophysiological Stress and EMG Activity of the Trapezius Muscle," *International Journal of Behavioral Medicine* 1, no. 4 (1994): 354–370, https://doi.org/10.1207/S15327558IJBM0104_5; Ioannis A. Pavlou et al., "Neurobiology of Bruxism: The Impact of Stress (Review)," Biomedical Reports 20, no. 4 (2024): 59, https://doi.org/10.3892/br.2024.1747..
[13] Johan W.S. Vlaeyen and Steven J. Linton, "Fear-Avoidance and Its Consequences in Chronic Musculoskeletal Pain: A State of the Art," *Pain* 85, no. 3 (April 2000): 317–32,
https://doi.org/10.1016/s0304-3959(99)00242-0.
[14] Temitayo Olugbade, Nadia Bianchi-Berthouze, and Amanda C de C. Williams, "The Relationship between Guarding, Pain, and Emotion," *PAIN Reports* 4, no. 4 (2019): e770,
https://www.ncbi.nlm.nih.gov/pmc/articles/PMC6728010/.
[15] Moseley, "A Pain Neuromatrix Approach to Patients with Chronic Pain."; Vlaeyen and Linton, "Fear-Avoidance and Its Consequences in Chronic Musculoskeletal Pain."
[16] Maaike Leeuw et al., "The Fear-Avoidance Model of Musculoskeletal Pain: Current State of Scientific Evidence," *Journal of Behavioral Medicine* 30, no. 1 (December 20, 2007): 77–94, https://doi.org/10.1007/s10865-006-9085-0.

Chapter 3

[1] Clifford J. Woolf, "Central Sensitization: Implications for the Diagnosis and Treatment of Pain," *Pain* 152, no. 3 (March 2011): S2–15,
https://doi.org/10.1016/j.pain.2010.09.030.
[2] G. Lorimer Moseley and David S. Butler, "Fifteen Years of Explaining Pain: The Past, Present, and Future," *The Journal of Pain* 16, no. 9 (September 2015): 807–13, https://doi.org/10.1016/j.jpain.2015.05.005.

[3] Ulf Lundberg et al., "Psychophysiological Stress and Emg Activity of the Trapezius Muscle," *International Journal of Behavioral Medicine* 1, no. 4 (December 1994): 354–70, https://doi.org/10.1207/s15327558ijbm0104_5.
[4] Andrea Zaccaro et al., "How Breath-Control Can Change Your Life: A Systematic Review on Psycho-Physiological Correlates of Slow Breathing," *Frontiers in Human Neuroscience* 12, no. 353 (September 7, 2018): 1–16, https://doi.org/10.3389/fnhum.2018.00353.
[5] Sara Magelssen Vambheim et al., "Relaxation Techniques as an Intervention for Chronic Pain: A Systematic Review of Randomized Controlled Trials," *Heliyon* 7, no. 8 (August 2021): e07837, https://doi.org/10.1016/j.heliyon.2021.e07837.
[6] Phil Page, "Current Concepts in Muscle Stretching for Exercise and Rehabilitation," *International Journal of Sports Physical Therapy* 7, no. 1 (February 1, 2012): 109–19, https://pubmed.ncbi.nlm.nih.gov/22319684/.
[7] C. H. Weppler and S. P. Magnusson, "Increasing Muscle Extensibility: A Matter of Increasing Length or Modifying Sensation?," *Physical Therapy* 90, no. 3 (January 14, 2010): 438–49, https://doi.org/10.2522/ptj.20090012.
[8] Uwe Proske and Simon C. Gandevia, "The Proprioceptive Senses: Their Roles in Signaling Body Shape, Body Position and Movement, and Muscle Force," *Physiological Reviews* 92, no. 4 (October 2012): 1651–97, https://doi.org/10.1152/physrev.00048.2011.
[9] Page, "Current Concepts in Muscle Stretching for Exercise and Rehabilitation."
[10] Carolyn Kisner, Lynn Allen Colby, and John Borstad, *Therapeutic Exercise: Foundations and Techniques*, 7th ed. (Philadelphia, PA: F.A. Davis Company, 2017).
[11] Sara Magelssen Vambheim, Tonje Merete Kyllo, Sanne Hegland, and Martin Bystad, "Relaxation Techniques as an Intervention for Chronic Pain: A Systematic Review of Randomized Controlled Trials," Heliyon 7, no. 8 (2021): e07837, https://doi.org/10.1016/j.heliyon.2021.e07837.
[12] Emma Meehan and Bernie Carter, "Moving with Pain: What Principles from Somatic Practices Can Offer to People Living with Chronic Pain," *Frontiers in Psychology* 11 (January 25, 2021), https://doi.org/10.3389/fpsyg.2020.620381.

[13] Weppler and Magnusson, "Increasing Muscle Extensibility."
[14] C.C. Streeter et al., "Effects of Yoga on the Autonomic Nervous System, Gamma-Aminobutyric-Acid, and Allostasis in Epilepsy, Depression, and Post-Traumatic Stress Disorder," *Medical Hypotheses* 78, no. 5 (May 2012): 571–79, https://doi.org/10.1016/j.mehy.2012.01.021; Michaela C. Pascoe and Isabelle E. Bauer, "A Systematic Review of Randomised Control Trials on the Effects of Yoga on Stress Measures and Mood," *Journal of Psychiatric Research* 68, no. 1 (September 2015): 270–82, https://doi.org/10.1016/j.jpsychires.2015.07.013.
[15] Streeter et al., "Effects of Yoga on the Autonomic Nervous System."; Zaccaro et al., "How Breath-Control Can Change Your Life."
[16] Sang-Dol Kim, "Yoga for Menstrual Pain in Primary Dysmenorrhea: A Meta-Analysis of Randomized Controlled Trials," *Complementary Therapies in Clinical Practice* 36 (August 2019): 94–99, https://doi.org/10.1016/j.ctcp.2019.06.006.
[17] Streeter et al., "Effects of Yoga on the Autonomic Nervous System."
[18] Lundberg et al., "Psychophysiological Stress and EMG Activity of the Trapezius Muscle."
[19] Vlaeyen and Linton, "Fear-Avoidance and Its Consequences in Chronic Musculoskeletal Pain."
[20] Moseley and Butler, "Fifteen Years of Explaining Pain."

Chapter 4

[1] Christopher T.V. Swain et al., "No Consensus on Causality of Spine Postures or Physical Exposure and Low Back Pain: A Systematic Review of Systematic Reviews," *Journal of Biomechanics* 102 (August 2019): 109312, https://doi.org/10.1016/j.jbiomech.2019.08.006; Ulrika Aasa et al., "Variability of Lumbar Spinal Alignment among Power- and Weightlifters during the Deadlift and Barbell Back Squat," *Sports Biomechanics*, November 13, 2019, 1–17, https://doi.org/10.1080/14763141.2019.1675751;
[2] Christopher T. V. Swain et al., "No Consensus on Causality of Spine Postures or Physical Exposure and Low Back Pain: A Systematic Review of Systematic Reviews," Journal of Biomechanics 102 (2020): 109312, https://doi.org/10.1016/j.jbiomech.2019.08.006.

[3] G. Lorimer Moseley and David S. Butler, "Fifteen Years of Explaining Pain: The Past, Present, and Future," *The Journal of Pain* 16, no. 9 (September 2015): 807–13, https://doi.org/10.1016/j.jpain.2015.05.005; Johan W.S. Vlaeyen and Steven J. Linton, "Fear-Avoidance and Its Consequences in Chronic Musculoskeletal Pain: A State of the Art," *Pain* 85, no. 3 (April 2000): 317–32, https://doi.org/10.1016/s0304-3959(99)00242-0.

[4] Lotte Veenstra, Iris K. Schneider, and Sander L. Koole, "Embodied Mood Regulation: The Impact of Body Posture on Mood Recovery, Negative Thoughts, and Mood-Congruent Recall," *Cognition and Emotion* 31, no. 7 (September 14, 2016): 1–16, https://doi.org/10.1080/02699931.2016.1225003.

[5] Christopher T.V. Swain et al., "No Consensus on Causality of Spine Postures or Physical Exposure and Low Back Pain: A Systematic Review of Systematic Reviews," *Journal of Biomechanics* 102 (August 2019): 109312, https://doi.org/10.1016/j.jbiomech.2019.08.006; D. Slater and P. O'Sullivan, "'Hands Off': Why Manual Therapy May Not Be the Most Effective Approach to Low Back Pain," British Journal of Sports Medicine 53, no. 19 (2019): 1239–40, https://doi.org/10.1136/bjsports-2018-100032.

[6] Moseley and Butler, "Fifteen Years of Explaining Pain," 807.

[7] Inge Timmers et al., "The Interaction between Stress and Chronic Pain through the Lens of Threat Learning," *Neuroscience & Biobehavioral Reviews* 107 (2019): 641–655, https://doi.org/10.1016/j.neubiorev.2019.10.007; Alejandro Luque-Suarez, Javier Martinez-Calderon, and Deborah Falla, "Role of Kinesiophobia on Pain, Disability and Quality of Life in People Suffering from Chronic Musculoskeletal Pain: A Systematic Review," *British Journal of Sports Medicine* 53, no. 9 (2019): 554–559, https://doi.org/10.1136/bjsports-2017-098673.

[8] Paul W. Hodges and G.Lorimer Moseley, "Pain and Motor Control of the Lumbopelvic Region: Effect and Possible Mechanisms," *Journal of Electromyography and Kinesiology* 13, no. 4 (August 2003): 361–70, https://doi.org/10.1016/s1050-6411(03)00042-7.

[9] Carolyn Kisner, Lynn A. Colby, and Janie Borstad, *Therapeutic Exercise: Foundations and Techniques*, 7th ed. (Philadelphia, PA: F.A. Davis Company, 2017).

Chapter 5

[1] James Steele, Stewart Bruce-Low, and Dave Smith, "A Review of the Specificity of Exercises Designed for Conditioning the Lumbar Extensors," *British Journal of Sports Medicine* 49, no. 5 (October 3, 2013): 291–97, https://doi.org/10.1136/bjsports-2013-092197.

[2] G. Lorimer Moseley and David S. Butler, "Fifteen Years of Explaining Pain: The Past, Present, and Future," *The Journal of Pain* 16, no. 9 (September 2015): 807–13, https://doi.org/10.1016/j.jpain.2015.05.005; Paul W. Hodges and G.Lorimer Moseley, "Pain and Motor Control of the Lumbopelvic Region: Effect and Possible Mechanisms," *Journal of Electromyography and Kinesiology* 13, no. 4 (August 2003): 361–70, https://doi.org/10.1016/s1050-6411(03)00042-7.

[3] Johan W.S. Vlaeyen and Steven J. Linton, "Fear-Avoidance and Its Consequences in Chronic Musculoskeletal Pain: A State of the Art," *Pain* 85, no. 3 (April 2000): 317–32, https://doi.org/10.1016/s0304-3959(99)00242-0; Patrick H. Finan, Burel R. Goodin, and Michael T. Smith, "The Association of Sleep and Pain: An Update and a Path Forward," *The Journal of Pain* 14, no. 12 (December 2013): 1539–52, https://doi.org/10.1016/j.jpain.2013.08.007.

[4] Johannes Blomgren et al., "Effects of Deep Cervical Flexor Training on Impaired Physiological Functions Associated with Chronic Neck Pain: A Systematic Review," *BMC Musculoskeletal Disorders* 19 (2018): 415, https://doi.org/10.1186/s12891-018-2324-z; Yong Gon Seo et al., "Is Scapular Stabilization Exercise Effective for Managing Nonspecific Chronic Neck Pain?: A Systematic Review," *Asian Spine Journal* 14, no. 1 (2020): 122–129, https://doi.org/10.31616/asj.2019.0125; Sean G. Sadler et al., "Gluteus Medius Muscle Function in People with and without Low Back Pain: A Systematic Review," *BMC Musculoskeletal Disorders* 20 (2019): 463, https://doi.org/10.1186/s12891-019-2833-4.

[5] Finan, Goodin, and Smith, "Association of Sleep and Pain," 1541; Vlaeyen and Linton, "Fear-Avoidance," 320.

[6] Moseley and Butler, "Fifteen Years of Explaining Pain," 810.

Chapter 6

[1] Dirk De Ridder, Divya Adhia, and Sven Vanneste, "The Anatomy of Pain and Suffering in the Brain and Its Clinical Implications," *Neuroscience & Biobehavioral Reviews* 130, no. 130 (November 2021): 125–46, https://doi.org/10.1016/j.neubiorev.2021.08.013; Johan W.S. Vlaeyen and Steven J. Linton, "Fear-Avoidance and Its Consequences in Chronic Musculoskeletal Pain: A State of the Art," *Pain* 85, no. 3 (April 2000): 317–32, https://doi.org/10.1016/s0304-3959(99)00242-0.
[2] Timmers et al., "The Interaction between Stress and Chronic Pain through the Lens of Threat Learning," Neuroscience & Biobehavioral Reviews 107 (December 2019): 641–655,
https://doi.org/10.1016/j.neubiorev.2019.10.007.
[3] Bruce S. McEwen, "Physiology and Neurobiology of Stress and Adaptation: Central Role of the Brain," *Physiological Reviews* 87, no. 3 (2007): 873–904, https://doi.org/10.1152/physrev.00041.2006.
[4] Stephen W. Porges, "The Polyvagal Perspective," *Biological Psychology* 74, no. 2 (February 2007): 116–43,
https://doi.org/10.1016/j.biopsycho.2006.06.009.
[5] Andrea Zaccaro et al., "How Breath-Control Can Change Your Life: A Systematic Review on Psycho-Physiological Correlates of Slow Breathing," *Frontiers in Human Neuroscience* 12, no. 353 (September 7, 2018): 1–16, https://doi.org/10.3389/fnhum.2018.00353; M. Kox et al., "Voluntary Activation of the Sympathetic Nervous System and Attenuation of the Innate Immune Response in Humans," *Proceedings of the National Academy of Sciences* 111, no. 20 (May 5, 2014): 7379–84,
https://doi.org/10.1073/pnas.1322174111.
[6] Stephen W. Porges, "The Polyvagal Perspective," *Biological Psychology* 74, no. 2 (2007): 116–143, https://doi.org/10.1016/j.biopsycho.2006.06.009; Wolf E. Mehling et al., "The Multidimensional Assessment of Interoceptive Awareness (MAIA)," ed. Manos Tsakiris, *PLoS ONE* 7, no. 11 (2012): e48230, https://doi.org/10.1371/journal.pone.0048230; Stephen M. Kosslyn, Giorgio Ganis, and William L. Thompson, "Neural Foundations of Imagery," *Nature Reviews Neuroscience* 2, no. 9 (2001): 635–642, https://doi.org/10.1038/35090055.
[7] Bessel van der Kolk, *The Body Keeps the Score: Brain, Mind and Body in the Healing of Trauma* (New York: Penguin Books, 2015).

[8] Temitayo Olugbade, Nadia Bianchi-Berthouze, and Amanda C de C. Williams, "The Relationship between Guarding, Pain, and Emotion," *PAIN Reports* 4, no. 4 (2019): e770, https://www.ncbi.nlm.nih.gov/pmc/articles/PMC6728010/.
[9] Eric L. Garland et al., "Mindfulness-Oriented Recovery Enhancement Reduces Opioid Dose in Primary Care by Strengthening Autonomic Regulation during Meditation.," *American Psychologist* 75, no. 6 (September 2020): 840–52, https://doi.org/10.1037/amp0000638; F. Zeidan et al., "Mindfulness Meditation-Related Pain Relief: Evidence for Unique Brain Mechanisms in the Regulation of Pain," *Neuroscience Letters* 520, no. 2 (June 2012): 165–73, https://doi.org/10.1016/j.neulet.2012.03.082.
[10] Garland et al., "Mindfulness-Oriented Recovery Enhancement," 845; Yi-Yuan Tang, Britta K. Hölzel, and Michael I. Posner, "The Neuroscience of Mindfulness Meditation," Nature Reviews Neuroscience 16, no. 4 (March 18, 2015): 213–25, https://doi.org/10.1038/nrn3916.
[11] McEwen, "Physiology and Neurobiology of Stress and Adaptation," 880.
[12] Andrea Zaccaro et al., "How Breath-Control Can Change Your Life: A Systematic Review on Psycho-Physiological Correlates of Slow Breathing," *Frontiers in Human Neuroscience* 12, no. 353 (September 7, 2018): 1–16, https://doi.org/10.3389/fnhum.2018.00353.
[13] McEwen, "Physiology and Neurobiology of Stress and Adaptation," 880; Van der Kolk, *The Body Keeps the Score*, 45.
[14] Sara Magelssen Vambheim et al., "Relaxation Techniques as an Intervention for Chronic Pain: A Systematic Review of Randomized Controlled Trials," *Heliyon* 7, no. 8 (August 2021): e07837, https://doi.org/10.1016/j.heliyon.2021.e07837.
[15] J David Creswell, "Mindfulness Interventions," *Annual Review of Psychology* 68, no. 1 (2017): 491–516, https://doi.org/10.1146/annurev-psych-042716-051139; Tang, Hölzel, and Posner, "The Neuroscience of Mindfulness Meditation."
[16] Timmers et al., "The Interaction between Stress and Chronic Pain through the Lens of Threat Learning."; Vambheim et al., "Relaxation Techniques as an Intervention for Chronic Pain."

Bibliography

Aasa, Ulrika, Victor Bengtsson, Lars Berglund, and Fredrik Öhberg. "Variability of Lumbar Spinal Alignment among Power- and Weightlifters during the Deadlift and Barbell Back Squat." *Sports Biomechanics*, November 13, 2019, 1–17. https://doi.org/10.1080/14763141.2019.1675751.

Apkarian, A. Vania, Marwan N. Baliki, and Paul Y. Geha. "Towards a Theory of Chronic Pain." *Progress in Neurobiology* 87, no. 2 (February 2009): 81–97. https://doi.org/10.1016/j.pneurobio.2008.09.018.

Bennie, Jason A, Josephine Y Chau, Hidde P van der Ploeg, Emmanuel Stamatakis, Anna Do, and Adrian Bauman. "The Prevalence and Correlates of Sitting in European Adults - a Comparison of 32 Eurobarometer-Participating Countries." *International Journal of Behavioral Nutrition and Physical Activity* 10, no. 1 (2013): 107. https://doi.org/10.1186/1479-5868-10-107.

Berg, W.B. van den. "Osteoarthritis Year 2010 in Review: Pathomechanisms." *Osteoarthritis and Cartilage* 19, no. 4 (April 2011): 338–41. https://doi.org/10.1016/j.joca.2011.01.022.

Biswas, Aviroop, Paul I. Oh, Guy E. Faulkner, Ravi R. Bajaj, Michael A. Silver, Marc S. Mitchell, and David A. Alter. "Sedentary Time and Its Association with Risk for Disease Incidence, Mortality, and Hospitalization in Adults." *Annals of Internal Medicine* 162, no. 2 (January 20, 2015): 123. https://doi.org/10.7326/m14-1651.

Booth, Frank W., Christian K. Roberts, and Matthew J. Laye. "Lack of Exercise Is a Major Cause of Chronic Diseases." *Comprehensive Physiology* 2, no. 2 (April 2012). https://doi.org/10.1002/cphy.c110025.

Chu, Brianna, Komal Marwaha, Derek Ayers, and Terrence Sanvictores. "Physiology, Stress Reaction." PubMed. Treasure Island (FL): StatPearls Publishing, May 7, 2024. https://www.ncbi.nlm.nih.gov/books/NBK541120/.

Craig, A. D. "How Do You Feel? Interoception: The Sense of the Physiological Condition of the Body." *Nature Reviews Neuroscience* 3, no. 8 (August 2002): 655–66. https://doi.org/10.1038/nrn894.

Creswell, J David. "Mindfulness Interventions." *Annual Review of Psychology* 68, no. 1 (2017): 491–516. https://doi.org/10.1146/annurev-psych-042716-051139.

De Ridder, Dirk, Divya Adhia, and Sven Vanneste. "The Anatomy of Pain and Suffering in the Brain and Its Clinical Implications." *Neuroscience & Biobehavioral Reviews* 130, no. 130 (November 2021): 125–46. https://doi.org/10.1016/j.neubiorev.2021.08.013.

Finan, Patrick H., Burel R. Goodin, and Michael T. Smith. "The Association of Sleep and Pain: An Update and a Path Forward." *The Journal of Pain* 14, no. 12 (December 2013): 1539–52. https://doi.org/10.1016/j.jpain.2013.08.007.

Flor, Herta, Christoph Braun, Thomas Elbert, and Niels Birbaumer. "Extensive Reorganization of Primary Somatosensory Cortex in Chronic Back Pain Patients." *Neuroscience Letters* 224, no. 1 (March 1997): 5–8. https://doi.org/10.1016/s0304-3940(97)13441-3.

Gabor Maté, MD. *When the Body Says No.* Vintage Canada, 2011.

Garland, Eric L., Justin Hudak, Adam W. Hanley, and Yoshio Nakamura. "Mindfulness-Oriented Recovery Enhancement Reduces Opioid Dose in Primary Care by Strengthening Autonomic Regulation during Meditation." *American Psychologist* 75, no. 6 (September 2020): 840–52. https://doi.org/10.1037/amp0000638.

Hodges, Paul W., and G.Lorimer Moseley. "Pain and Motor Control of the Lumbopelvic Region: Effect and Possible Mechanisms." *Journal of Electromyography and Kinesiology* 13, no. 4 (August 2003): 361–70. https://doi.org/10.1016/s1050-6411(03)00042-7.

International Association for the Study of Pain. "Terminology." International Association for the Study of Pain (IASP), 2020. https://www.iasp-pain.org/resources/terminology/.

Jull, G. "Management of Cervical Headache." *Manual Therapy* 2, no. 4 (November 1997): 182–90. https://doi.org/10.1054/math.1997.0298.

Kibler, W. Ben, J.O.H.N. McMullen, and T.I.M. UHL. "Shoulder Rehabilitation Strategies, Guidelines, and Practice." *Orthopedic Clinics of North America* 32, no. 3 (July 2001): 527–38. https://doi.org/10.1016/s0030-5898(05)70222-4.

Kim, Sang-Dol. "Yoga for Menstrual Pain in Primary Dysmenorrhea: A Meta-Analysis of Randomized Controlled Trials." *Complementary Therapies in Clinical Practice* 36 (August 2019): 94–99. https://doi.org/10.1016/j.ctcp.2019.06.006.

Kolk, Bessel van der. *The Body Keeps the Score: Brain, Mind and Body in the Healing of Trauma*. New York: Penguin Books, 2015.

Kox, M., L. T. van Eijk, J. Zwaag, J. van den Wildenberg, F. C. G. J. Sweep, J. G. van der Hoeven, and P. Pickkers. "Voluntary Activation of the Sympathetic Nervous System and Attenuation of the Innate Immune Response in Humans." *Proceedings of the National Academy of Sciences* 111, no. 20 (May 5, 2014): 7379–84. https://doi.org/10.1073/pnas.1322174111.

Leeuw, Maaike, Mariëlle E. J. B. Goossens, Steven J. Linton, Geert Crombez, Katja Boersma, and Johan W. S. Vlaeyen. "The Fear-Avoidance Model of Musculoskeletal Pain: Current State of Scientific Evidence." *Journal of Behavioral Medicine* 30, no. 1 (December 20, 2007): 77–94. https://doi.org/10.1007/s10865-006-9085-0.

Louw, Adriaan, Kory Zimney, Emilio J. Puentedura, and Ina Diener. "The Efficacy of Pain Neuroscience Education on Musculoskeletal Pain: A Systematic Review of the Literature." *Physiotherapy Theory and Practice* 32, no. 5 (June 28, 2016): 332–55. https://doi.org/10.1080/09593985.2016.1194646.

Lundberg, Ulf, Roland Kadefors, Bo Melin, Gunnar Palmerud, Peter Hassmén, Margareta Engström, and Ingela Elfsberg Dohns. "Psychophysiological Stress and Emg Activity of the Trapezius Muscle." *International Journal of Behavioral Medicine* 1, no. 4 (December 1994): 354–70. https://doi.org/10.1207/s15327558ijbm0104_5.

Martin, Paul R. "Behavioral Management of Migraine Headache Triggers: Learning to Cope with Triggers." *Current Pain and Headache Reports* 14, no. 3 (April 27, 2010): 221–27. https://doi.org/10.1007/s11916-010-0112-z.

McEwen, Bruce S. "Physiology and Neurobiology of Stress and Adaptation: Central Role of the Brain." *Physiological Reviews* 87, no. 3 (2007): 873–904. https://doi.org/10.1152/physrev.00041.2006.

Meehan, Emma, and Bernie Carter. "Moving with Pain: What Principles from Somatic Practices Can Offer to People Living with Chronic Pain." *Frontiers in Psychology* 11 (January 25, 2021). https://doi.org/10.3389/fpsyg.2020.620381.

Mehling, Wolf E., Cynthia Price, Jennifer J. Daubenmier, Mike Acree, Elizabeth Bartmess, and Anita Stewart. "The Multidimensional Assessment of Interoceptive Awareness (MAIA)." Edited by

Manos Tsakiris. *PLoS ONE* 7, no. 11 (November 1, 2012): e48230. https://doi.org/10.1371/journal.pone.0048230.

Moseley, G. Lorimer, and David S. Butler. "Fifteen Years of Explaining Pain: The Past, Present, and Future." *The Journal of Pain* 16, no. 9 (September 2015): 807–13. https://doi.org/10.1016/j.jpain.2015.05.005.

Moseley, G. Lorimer, and Herta Flor. "Targeting Cortical Representations in the Treatment of Chronic Pain." *Neurorehabilitation and Neural Repair* 26, no. 6 (February 13, 2012): 646–52. https://doi.org/10.1177/1545968311433209.

Moseley, G.L. "A Pain Neuromatrix Approach to Patients with Chronic Pain." *Manual Therapy* 8, no. 3 (August 2003): 130–40. https://doi.org/10.1016/s1356-689x(03)00051-1.

Olugbade, Temitayo, Nadia Bianchi-Berthouze, and Amanda C de C. Williams. "The Relationship between Guarding, Pain, and Emotion." *PAIN Reports* 4, no. 4 (2019): e770. https://www.ncbi.nlm.nih.gov/pmc/articles/PMC6728010/.

Osterweis, Marian, Arthur Kleinman, and David Mechanic. "The Anatomy and Physiology of Pain." National Library of Medicine. National Academies Press (US), 1987. https://www.ncbi.nlm.nih.gov/books/NBK219252/.

Page, Phil. "Current Concepts in Muscle Stretching for Exercise and Rehabilitation." *International Journal of Sports Physical Therapy* 7, no. 1 (February 1, 2012): 109–19. https://pubmed.ncbi.nlm.nih.gov/22319684/.

Pascoe, Michaela C., and Isabelle E. Bauer. "A Systematic Review of Randomised Control Trials on the Effects of Yoga on Stress Measures and Mood." *Journal of Psychiatric Research* 68, no. 1 (September 2015): 270–82. https://doi.org/10.1016/j.jpsychires.2015.07.013.

Porges, Stephen W. "The Polyvagal Perspective." *Biological Psychology* 74, no. 2 (February 2007): 116–43. https://doi.org/10.1016/j.biopsycho.2006.06.009.

Proske, Uwe, and Simon C. Gandevia. "The Proprioceptive Senses: Their Roles in Signaling Body Shape, Body Position and Movement, and Muscle Force." *Physiological Reviews* 92, no. 4 (October 2012): 1651–97. https://doi.org/10.1152/physrev.00048.2011.

Rayane Haddadj, Anne Lovise Nordstoga, Tom Ivar, Eivind Schjelderup Skarpsno, Atle Kongsvold, Mats Flaaten, Jasper Schipperijn, Kerstin Bach, and Paul Jarle Mork. "Volume and Intensity of

Walking and Risk of Chronic Low Back Pain." *JAMA Network Open* 8, no. 6 (June 13, 2025): e2515592–92. https://doi.org/10.1001/jamanetworkopen.2025.15592.

Santos, Erick Alves dos, Beatriz Rodrigues Risuenho Peinado, Deborah Ribeiro Frazão, Yago Gecy de Sousa Né, Nathalia Carolina Fernandes Fagundes, Marcela Baraúna Magno, Lucianne Cople Maia, Rafael Rodrigues Lima, and Renata Duarte de Souza-Rodrigues. "Association between Temporomandibular Disorders and Anxiety: A Systematic Review." *Frontiers in Psychiatry* 13 (October 13, 2022). https://doi.org/10.3389/fpsyt.2022.990430.

Steele, James, Stewart Bruce-Low, and Dave Smith. "A Review of the Specificity of Exercises Designed for Conditioning the Lumbar Extensors." *British Journal of Sports Medicine* 49, no. 5 (October 3, 2013): 291–97. https://doi.org/10.1136/bjsports-2013-092197.

Streeter, C.C., P.L. Gerbarg, R.B. Saper, D.A. Ciraulo, and R.P. Brown. "Effects of Yoga on the Autonomic Nervous System, Gamma-Aminobutyric-Acid, and Allostasis in Epilepsy, Depression, and Post-Traumatic Stress Disorder." *Medical Hypotheses* 78, no. 5 (May 2012): 571–79. https://doi.org/10.1016/j.mehy.2012.01.021.

Stults-Kolehmainen, Matthew A. "Humans Have a Basic Physical and Psychological Need to Move the Body: Physical Activity as a Primary Drive." *Frontiers in Psychology* 14 (April 11, 2023). https://doi.org/10.3389/fpsyg.2023.1134049.

Swain, Christopher T.V., Fumin Pan, Patrick J. Owen, Hendrik Schmidt, and Daniel L. Belavy. "No Consensus on Causality of Spine Postures or Physical Exposure and Low Back Pain: A Systematic Review of Systematic Reviews." *Journal of Biomechanics* 102 (August 2019): 109312. https://doi.org/10.1016/j.jbiomech.2019.08.006.

Tang, Yi-Yuan, Britta K. Hölzel, and Michael I. Posner. "The Neuroscience of Mindfulness Meditation." *Nature Reviews Neuroscience* 16, no. 4 (March 18, 2015): 213–25. https://doi.org/10.1038/nrn3916.

Timmers, Inge, Conny W.E.M. Quaedflieg, Connie Hsu, Lauren C. Heathcote, Cynthia R. Rovnaghi, and Laura E. Simons. "The Interaction between Stress and Chronic Pain through the Lens of Threat Learning." *Neuroscience & Biobehavioral Reviews* 107, no. 1 (December 2019): 641–55. https://doi.org/10.1016/j.neubiorev.2019.10.007.

Traeger, Adrian C., Markus Hübscher, Nicholas Henschke, G. Lorimer Moseley, Hopin Lee, and James H. McAuley. "Effect of Primary Care–Based Education on Reassurance in Patients with Acute

Low Back Pain: Systematic Review and Meta-Analysis." *JAMA Internal Medicine* 175, no. 5 (May 1, 2015): 733–43. https://doi.org/10.1001/jamainternmed.2015.0217.

Treleaven, Julia. "Sensorimotor Disturbances in Neck Disorders Affecting Postural Stability, Head and Eye Movement Control." *Manual Therapy* 13, no. 1 (February 2008): 2–11. https://doi.org/10.1016/j.math.2007.06.003.

Veenstra, Lotte, Iris K. Schneider, and Sander L. Koole. "Embodied Mood Regulation: The Impact of Body Posture on Mood Recovery, Negative Thoughts, and Mood-Congruent Recall." *Cognition and Emotion 31*, no. 7 (September 14, 2016): 1–16. https://doi.org/10.1080/02699931.2016.1225003.

Vambheim, Sara Magelssen, Tonje Merete Kyllo, Sanne Hegland, and Martin Bystad. "Relaxation Techniques as an Intervention for Chronic Pain: A Systematic Review of Randomized Controlled Trials." *Heliyon* 7, no. 8 (August 2021): e07837. https://doi.org/10.1016/j.heliyon.2021.e07837.

Vergroesen, P.-P.A., I. Kingma, K.S. Emanuel, R.J.W. Hoogendoorn, T.J. Welting, B.J. van Royen, J.H. van Dieën, and T.H. Smit. "Mechanics and Biology in Intervertebral Disc Degeneration: A Vicious Circle." *Osteoarthritis and Cartilage* 23, no. 7 (July 2015): 1057–70. https://doi.org/10.1016/j.joca.2015.03.028.

Vlaeyen, Johan W.S., and Steven J. Linton. "Fear-Avoidance and Its Consequences in Chronic Musculoskeletal Pain: A State of the Art." *Pain* 85, no. 3 (April 2000): 317–32. https://doi.org/10.1016/s0304-3959(99)00242-0.

Weppler, C. H., and S. P. Magnusson. "Increasing Muscle Extensibility: A Matter of Increasing Length or Modifying Sensation?" *Physical Therapy* 90, no. 3 (January 14, 2010): 438–49. https://doi.org/10.2522/ptj.20090012.

Wiech, K. "Deconstructing the Sensation of Pain: The Influence of Cognitive Processes on Pain Perception." *Science* 354, no. 6312 (November 3, 2016): 584–87. https://doi.org/10.1126/science.aaf8934.

Williams, P E, and G Goldspink. "Connective Tissue Changes in Immobilised Muscle." *Journal of Anatomy* 138, no. Pt 2 (March 1984): 343. https://pmc.ncbi.nlm.nih.gov/articles/PMC1164074/.

Woolf, Clifford J. "Central Sensitization: Implications for the Diagnosis and Treatment of Pain." *Pain* 152, no. 3 (March 2011): S2–15. https://doi.org/10.1016/j.pain.2010.09.030.

Zaccaro, Andrea, Andrea Piarulli, Marco Laurino, Erika Garbella, Danilo Menicucci, Bruno Neri, and Angelo Gemignani. "How Breath-Control Can Change Your Life: A Systematic Review on Psycho-Physiological Correlates of Slow Breathing." *Frontiers in Human Neuroscience* 12, no. 353 (September 7, 2018): 1–16. https://doi.org/10.3389/fnhum.2018.00353.

Zale, Emily L, and Joseph W Ditre. "Pain-Related Fear, Disability, and the Fear-Avoidance Model of Chronic Pain." *Current Opinion in Psychology* 5, no. 5 (October 2015): 24–30. https://doi.org/10.1016/j.copsyc.2015.03.014.

Zeidan, F., J.A. Grant, C.A. Brown, J.G. McHaffie, and R.C. Coghill. "Mindfulness Meditation-Related Pain Relief: Evidence for Unique Brain Mechanisms in the Regulation of Pain." *Neuroscience Letters* 520, no. 2 (June 2012): 165–73. https://doi.org/10.1016/j.neulet.2012.03.082.

www.ingramcontent.com/pod-product-compliance
Lightning Source LLC
LaVergne TN
LVHW010721061126
851857LV00014B/1297
* 9 7 8 9 6 1 9 7 4 0 1 1 8 *